"What a gift to the Yoga community! This book is t    revolutionary indeed. Practical, raw, and real. Thro           ...yman makes the philosophy livable and the practices doable for everybody."—INDU ARORA, author of *Yoga* and *Mudra*

"In *Yoga Revolution*, Jivana Heyman leads us into the truth of the ancient practice of yoga, which is above all to love and serve humanity—and he gives us the tools to do so. By sharing his own stories so freely—and passing along what he has learned on the path—he encourages us all to discover for ourselves how we can use yoga, in some small way, to ease the suffering in the world."—LINDA SPARROWE, former editor-in-chief of *Yoga International* and author of *Yoga Mama*

"Our culture is very good at shutting people and conversations down. What I appreciate most about this book is that it is designed to promote deep and thoughtful conversation about yoga and to open spaces of dialogue, learning, and healing. I can't wait to talk with others about it!"—JEREMY DAVID ENGELS, author of *The Ethics of Oneness*

"*Yoga Revolution* is a critical call to action for yoga professionals and practitioners alike."—MATTHEW J. TAYLOR, PT, PhD, C-IAYT, past president of the International Association of Yoga Therapists

"With depth of understanding and clarity of reason, Jivana Heyman reminds us that it's both possible and important to hold past and present—evolution and revolution—in the same breath. Swami Rama once said that we must remember that we are simultaneously citizens of two worlds—the inner world and the outer world. This book helps anchor us in our inner world as we commit to the serious work of the outer. Reading *Yoga Revolution* left me both informed and inspired. I am deeply grateful."—NIKKI MYERS, founder of Yoga of 12-Step Recovery

"A heartfelt reminder that yoga is not about us but a much bigger picture. Although early yogis withdrew from the world to seek spiritual truth, blissing out in a bubble means ignoring injustice. As Jivana Heyman persuasively argues in *Yoga Revolution*, a more balanced approach is to care for ourselves so that we're better resourced to serve others." —DANIEL SIMPSON, author of *The Truth of Yoga*

"This book is a deeply personal integration of the spiritual principles of yoga presented in an utterly relevant and engaging format. I was touched by the numerous stories that Jivana shared, as well as by the yoga teacher profiles. A great effort has been made here to process the traditional Indian origins of yoga in a contemporary social and cultural context. This is a teaching every yoga student in the US should certainly read!" —KINO MACGREGOR, author of *Get Your Yoga On*

"*Yoga Revolution* is a love song to the practice of yoga. What a blessing and a gift to us all." —MELANIE KLEIN, author of *Embodied Resilience through Yoga*

"*Yoga Revolution* is an indispensable guide for all contemporary practitioners striving to respect the roots of the yoga tradition while using the practice to guide comprehensive social change."—JASON CRANDELL, Vinyasa teacher, contributor to *Yoga Journal*

"Yoga is much more than asana, and this book explores the intersection of yoga and social justice as a vehicle for revolution internally and externally, which is much needed globally in the time we are in"—ANUSHA WIJEYAKUMAR, MA, CPC, E-RYT, author of *Meditation with Intention*

"Jivana has given us the gift of his heart and vulnerability as he invites us to look into the intersections of our yoga practice, activism, and commitment to social justice without abandoning ourselves. He toes the delicate balance of inviting us to hold grief and joy at the same time, to honor the non-linear journey of healing, and to lean into tools that allow us to show up more fully alive for the work we do. A must read for every yoga teacher."—ZAHABIYAH (ZABIE) YAMASAKI, MEd, RYT, author of *Trauma-Informed Yoga for Survivors of Sexual Assault*

"*Yoga Revolution* is exactly the book we need right now. Jivana addresses head on the way that spiritual practices like yoga can be harmful and superficial if not practiced with justice in mind, and—more importantly—he outlines how each of us can help in creating a much-needed revolution!"—HALA KHOURI, MA, author of *Peace from Anxiety*

"Through the layers of wisdom revealed in *Yoga Revolution*, readers have an opportunity to step into the light of activism and service for the greater good of all of humanity. This book is rich with wonderful personal stories and ancient teachings that are sure to illuminate readers' hearts."—CHERI CLAMPETT, C-IAYT, co-author of *The Therapeutic Yoga Kit*

"Jivana does a remarkable job of uplifting important source texts and using them to guide and support us in important modern social justice questions and inquiries. He acknowledges harm within yoga lineages, discusses current racial justice issues as yogic questions, and explains how systemic inequities come to bear on modern postural practice—shadows rarely explored by many yoga teachers and leaders. He presents the possibilities and the obstacles and the grief and the joy so thoroughly that I am compelled to dedicate even more to practice and to meet Jivana there as a comrade and spiritual friend."—JACOBY BALLARD, author of *A Queer Dharma*

"I am pleased to say that there is a yoga revolution where a worldwide community of teachers and students are coming together to help ensure that yoga is accessible and inclusive and available for everyone. I believe that this is an important and much-needed book to help us have a greater understanding of yoga."—DONNA NOBLE, founder the Noble Art of Yoga

"*Yoga Revolution* unites ancient teachings with a modern call for social justice and equity. Jivana revisits texts often used to bypass collective responsibility through an anti-oppression framework that instead upholds it. This book is ideal for teachers, aspiring teachers, and anyone wanting to deepen their yoga practice and contribute to community wellbeing."—BO FORBES, PsyD, author of *Yoga for Emotional Balance*

"With wisdom and knowledge, Jivana guides us through yoga from the ancient to the contemporary. Thank you, Jivana, for *Yoga Revolution*; it has inspired me to live my yoga

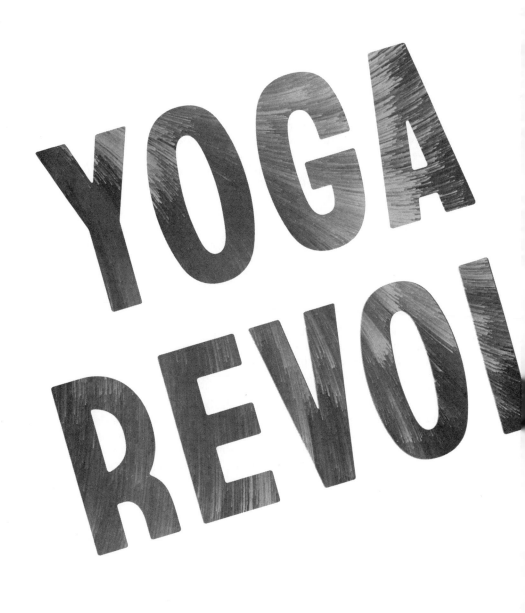

out loud!"—MAYA BREUER, VP Cross-Cultural Advancement, Yoga Alliance/Yoga Alliance Foundation

"*Yoga Revolution* is a gift to the yoga community, and it is also a necessary call to action. Jivana Heyman contextualizes the teachings of yoga in a way that exceeds any other attempt I've seen to date. He asks the tough questions while also demonstrating a tremendous amount of care and compassion for the reader. This book is exactly what the yoga world needs."—KAT (HEAGBERG) REBAR, author of *Yoga Where You Are* and editor-in-chief of *Yoga International*

"*Yoga Revolution* is a timely, personal, and deeply moving book, offering an applied yoga philosophy for the modern-day, socially-engaged practitioner. Drawing on his decades of personal study, practice, teaching, and activism, Jivana's work bravely combines the Gītā's call for *loka-saṃgraha*—the welfare of the world—with a compassionate vision of yoga that is truly accessible to all."— SETH POWELL (Harvard University), founder and director of Yogic Studies

"This book voices a dream and a hope for what the practice can be, and one shared by a growing movement of teachers, writers and practitioners—many of whose voices are also included. This is a beloved community in action, and one I am honored to find myself a part of."—THEO WILDCROFT, author of *Post-lineage Yoga*

"In this passionate and inspiring book, Jivana challenges us to change the way we think about and practice yoga. Rather than just focusing on cultivating equanimity or wellness, he shows us how to use yoga to fuel our compassion for others and to support us as we engage in acts of service and social activism while working to create a world that reflects yoga's message of unity, equity, and justice. This way of applying yoga's precepts and practices enables us to respond wholeheartedly to the difficulties of life in the modern world while at the same time respecting the roots of ancient yoga."—NINA ZOLOTOW, author of *Yoga for Healthy Aging* and *Yoga for Times of Change*

"Jivana Heyman's work in the world teaches us that healing lies in connection with others, with self-care as the first step in, and then stepping up to serve others. This is the quiet yet powerful revolution of yoga."—KALLIE SCHUT, founder of Rebel Yoga Tribe

"In a time when the world is experiencing revolutions on multiple fronts, it is only natural that the yoga community would find itself in a revolution of its own. This is a fascinating, groundbreaking book that offers practitioners a playbook by which 'we can allow yoga to reveal the truth of our own mind and heart.' *Yoga Revolution* is essential reading."—DR. TERRY HARRIS, co-founder and instructor at The Collective STL

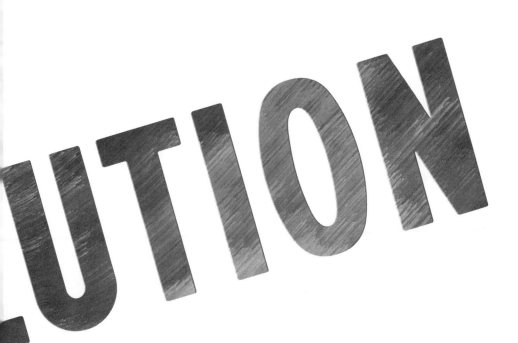

# Building a Practice of Courage and Compassion

JIVANA HEYMAN

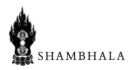

SHAMBHALA

Shambhala Publications, Inc.
2129 13th Street
Boulder, Colorado 80302
www.shambhala.com

The content of this book is not intended as medical advice. Please seek approval from your health care practitioner before attempting any of the methods described here.

Cover art: agsandrew / Shutterstock.com
Cover and interior design: Kate E. White

"Call Me By My True Names" by Thich Nhat Hanh. 2001.
Reprinted with permission from Parallax Press.
"A Cushion for Your Head," from the Penguin publication *The Gift: Poems by Hafiz* by Daniel Ladinsky, copyright 1999, and used with permission.
"The Failure" by Kabir and "The Jar with the Dry Rim" by Rumi from *The Soul is Here for Its Own Joy* edited and translated by Robert Bly. Copyright © 1995 by Robert Bly. Reprinted by permission of Georges Borchardt, Inc., for Robert Bly.

9 8 7 6 5 4 3 2 1

First Edition
Printed in the United States of America

♾ This edition is printed on acid-free paper that meets the
American National Standards Institute z39.48 Standard.
♻ Shambhala Publications makes every effort to print on recycled paper.
For more information please visit www.shambhala.com.
Shambhala Publications is distributed worldwide by
Penguin Random House, Inc., and its subsidiaries.

LIBRARY OF CONGRESS CATALOGING-IN-PUBLICATION DATA
Names: Heyman, Jivana, author.
Title: Yoga revolution: building a practice of courage and compassion / Jivana Heyman.
Description: First edition. | Boulder, Colorado: Shambhala Publications Inc., [2021]
Identifiers: LCCN 2021009395 | ISBN 9781611808780 (trade paperback)
Subjects: LCSH: Yoga.
Classification: LCC B132.Y6 H465 2021 | DDC 181/.45—dc23
LC record available at https://lccn.loc.gov/2021009395

## DEDICATION

For Matt, with love

# CONTENTS

X |

# FOREWORD

The first few times I ever talked with anyone about yoga or stepped into a class space I did not understand what I was being invited to experience. My socialization around movement, culture, and belonging said that the practice did not have a place in my experience, that I did not deserve it. The story that led my framed understanding of yoga said that the practice belonged to thin, rich, able-bodied women. I remember being a twenty-something flight attendant, barely able to afford my basic needs. I was physically and emotionally tired as I sat across from another flight attendant named Patty. She asked me if I had ever done yoga when she noticed I was reading Hermann Hesse's *Siddhartha*. I told her with absolute certainty that "Black people do not do yoga." In the more than fifteen years since, I have thought about that conversation often because Patty said something I know to be true now: this practice is for everyone.

When I finally made it into a welcoming and inviting yoga class, I was fortunate to find a teacher who would explain that yoga was more than a fitness program. And since that time I have been fortunate to find teachers along the way who expanded not only how I view the practice but have also invited me to see it as a way to create a more just and equitable world. In that fifteen years since my conversation with Patty, I have learned that the understanding that I had, that so many people have, of this practice being something that belongs to a privileged, dominant culture, is not by accident. The way that this sacred practice has been appropriated and turned into a billion-dollar industry is a purposeful display of white supremacy and its brainchild, capitalism. The practice has been marketed to us all as an exclusive luxury of a hippie lifestyle instead of the centuries-old philosophical life path I now know it to be. That appropriation has meant an erasure of the indigenous cultures that developed these rituals, practices, and texts. It has also meant reinterpretation of the texts, philosophies, and practices to uphold dominant culture, promote individualism, and enable white silence in the face of oppression.

About six years ago I began conversations about equity, representation, and community with longtime and well-known teachers within the yoga community in my hometown of Charlotte, North Carolina. I was a fairly new yoga teacher and feeling frustrated by the all-white studios and harmful community interactions. Frequently, the philosophy of this practice, the sacred texts, and the spaces were weaponized against those of us speaking up, asking for accountability, and seeking change. It has been frequently leveled at those of us who speak up that if we are truly doing this practice, the frustration, anger, and inaccessibility we see would disappear.

It has been tough to find teachers with platforms and enough perspective to see the connections between our social responsibility and this sacred practice. In many ways the community that has developed around this practice, in its current model, is willing to uphold white supremacy even inside of something that should be available to all. The spiritual and energetic parts of this practice have been removed, just like the Black and Brown people who developed it. For a large portion of those three years I have felt the pull of hopelessness that there is no use pushing for change.

Right now we are in a pivotal moment. The climate for change is aided by a pandemic, the use of social media to rally folks for change, and the rise of teachers within our community who are standing up for truth. We are blessed in this moment to have an emerging group of teachers who are stepping forward and supporting more equity and accessibility in a sustainable way. Jivana has been connected to that work for a while. The work he has led with Accessible Yoga has taught me so much and inspired me to lean into my own service. I am grateful to have met Jivana and to be in regular collaboration regarding equity and accessibility. As a Black, Queer person in a bigger body I am grateful for Jivana's early HIV advocacy and the space he creates to uplift voices like mine. His first book, *Accessible Yoga*, has become a go-to text for me, and I have similar gratitude for this new work from Jivana. The time of Black, LGBTQ, fat, and disabled teachers, students, and advocates being silenced is coming to an end, because we are done being silenced, ignored, and excluded.

What you are holding in your hands is an invitation to discover the ways we have contributed to keeping yoga practice for everyone. Jivana has given us a gift that asks us to truly understand the connections between our social action and this powerful spiritual modality. With compassion and clarity, Jivana makes plain how this practice actually requires us to be responsible for the greater world through deliberate social action. Using the same texts that have often been used to hide, bypass, and gaslight those demanding change, Jivana is lending a voice to the growing chorus of yogis speaking up for justice and highlighting how the practice supports it all.

—KELLEY PALMER

# ACKNOWLEDGMENTS

I need to begin with gratitude. How lucky I am to even get the chance to sit here and write—to explore my experiences and my practice in this way. It's a huge privilege that many people don't have. I appreciate this opportunity to explore yoga with you, and I'm grateful to you for reading. This book is about living the teachings—which manifest as service—and service begins with love and gratitude.

I want to thank my children, Charlie and Violet. They have been very patient with me as I pursue my dream of teaching and writing. I pray that I am an example of service to them, and not simply an example of workaholism. My hope is that they find a calling in life that fills them up as much as yoga has filled me.

I also want to mention my father, Ken Heyman, who died last year and was such an inspiration to me. He was a powerful artist who saw so much beauty in the world, and whose footsteps I'm trying to follow in. I encourage you to look up his photography and enjoy his beautiful vision of the world and the way he explored our shared humanity. His clear vision trained me to see the world in a particular way, and this book is my effort to share that with you.

Thank you to Swami Satchidananda and all my teachers. I had the gift of spending about eleven years studying with Swami Satchidananda in person and then later with most of his senior disciples. His approach to yoga made the teachings accessible for me, and his translations of Patanjali's Yoga Sutras and the Bhagavad Gita guide my understanding of these texts.

My main source of inspiration is the community of Accessible Yoga teachers and ambassadors all around the world and yoga teachers everywhere who are sharing yoga with their heart and soul. There is literally an army of peaceful warriors spreading love around the world through the practice of yoga. Most of these teachers go unacknowledged. They teach in yoga studios, gyms, community centers, prisons, hospitals, hospices, offices, schools, and anywhere people are looking for peace. This yoga army is fulfilling the vision of Krishna in the Bhagavad Gita and offering yoga as their service in the world. This book is for you, and you know who you are (although we may need a secret handshake).

I can't say enough good things about working with Sarit Z. Rogers, and how getting photographed by her relaxes me! I'm especially grateful to Kelley Palmer for writing the foreword, and for her friendship and unending wisdom. I also feel incredibly grateful to be working so closely with Amber Karnes, who constantly inspires me and challenges me. A shout-out goes to my fellow yoga teacher/friends who are included here as contributors. A detailed list of this incredible group, with information about their work, is included at the back of the book. I'm so grateful to them for sharing their words and practice with me and allowing me to share it with you.

I have been greatly influenced by a number of teachers and writers who have been writing about the intersection of yoga and social justice for some time. I want to acknowledge them and encourage you to study their work directly. This includes Michelle Cassandra Johnson, Susanna Barkataki, Dianne Bondy, Kat Rebar, Melanie Klein, Matthew Sanford, Kerri Kelly, Octavia Raheem, Hala Khouri, Theo Wildcroft, Kimberly Dark, Matthew Remski, Seane Corn, Linda Sparrowe, Lama Rod Owens, Michael Stone, and many others.

Thank you to the staff of Accessible Yoga, who are so dedicated to this work: Brina Lord, M Camellia, Tiph Browne, Deanna Michalopoulos, Sevika Ford, Garrett Jurss, Sarah Nuttridge, and Robyn Bell, and to our board: Amber Karnes, Pamela Stokes Eggleston, Mary Sims, Matthew Taylor, Amina Naru, Ashley Williams, Sarani Fedman, Priya Wagner, Tristan Katz, Anjali Rao, Colin Lieu, and previous member, Prashanti Goodell.

Special thanks to my editor, Beth Frankl, whom I have come to rely on completely (I'll have to write another book just to keep talking to her!), Samantha Ripley, Cannon Labrie, and all the staff at Shambhala for their grace and service to the world. I also want to thank *Yoga Journal* and *Yoga International*, where small snippets of this book first showed signs of life. A big thank-you to Nina Zolotow for all her support and important questions. I am so grateful to Daniel Simpson for his essential feedback. M Camellia, thank you for your insight and support with this book and all my projects!

Gratitude to my teachers and friends, Cheri Clampett, Matt Pesendian, David Lipsius, Swami Ramananda, Shannon Crow, Maitreyi Picerno, Seth Powell, and so many others.

Thank you for reading this book, and for being open to my vision of the yoga teachings. I hope you can find something useful here, and that it might plant a seed in your heart from which something beautiful will grow.

# INTRODUCTION

Modern yoga is finally growing up, and the time has come to address the dissonance between the superficial way yoga is currently being practiced and the depth of yoga's ancient universal spiritual teachings. Yoga offers so much more than fancy poses. At its core, yoga is a pathway to personal and community liberation, although traditionally it was more inwardly focused. It offers enlightenment—true independence—but not in the limited way we have been trained to conceptualize it.

I hope to share a new vision of what enlightenment looks like now. It's a state of mind that's expansive, open, and accepting—the result of an inner yoga revolution. A mind and a heart that are loving and compassionate and have the courage to be dedicated to service and social justice for all beings. A mind that sees itself in others and understands that the goals of yoga are only accomplished when we all have peace, justice, and equality—an outer revolution. That's the beauty of this practice, it calls for both an inner and outer transformation.

After decades of practice, I feel like I've finally reconciled my yoga practice with my activism, and I've found the shared root of both: love and compassion. I see that there is no separation between the personal and the political, and in practice, yoga takes the form of service and social justice. Our personal liberation is tied up with the liberation of our entire community, in the liberation of all beings. It's time to let go of the image of a yogi meditating alone in a cave divorced from society, and examine the way we are practicing right now and the way it impacts not only ourselves but the community around us.

Our yoga practice isn't going to solve the ills of the world—I realize that. But we can allow yoga to reveal the truth of our own mind and heart. We can allow our heart to expand with compassion for those who are suffering, starting with ourselves. In fact, if we are the ones suffering and feeling disempowered, we can use yoga for self-care and empowerment. Or, if we have privilege, we can allow yoga to expand our thinking to reveal the ways that we are benefiting from the inequities in society. Either way, yoga can support us in stepping up or stepping back, if we engage with our practice effectively.

We can't pick yoga apart and only use the physical practices without understanding their meaning and context. Instead, we need to look at how the philosophy of yoga speaks to the challenge of our contemporary society and the pressing issues that we face. In particular, we need to open our eyes to the ravages of white supremacy in all its many names and forms: racism, ableism, environmental degradation, xenophobia, ageism, homophobia, sexism, transphobia, fatphobia, and so on. These all represent what yoga is not.

This connection between the personal and the political is generally overlooked in contemporary yoga communities, taking the form of spiritual bypassing. It is another incarnation of white supremacy that allows those with privilege to use indigenous practices without consideration or compassion—without concern for others. Personally, I'm interested in finding a way to practice yoga that is respectful of tradition and still appropriate to this moment. It's a balancing act that relies on constant learning and humility. This book is an effort to learn as much as to teach, and I hope you are open to learning along with me.

My first book, *Accessible Yoga*, was inspired by the death of so many close friends to AIDS as well as my work sharing yoga with people with disabilities over the last twenty-five years of teaching. *Yoga Revolution* is the reconciliation of my AIDS activism with my yoga teaching in the time of Black Lives Matter—a cultural revolution. It's also a product of the struggles of my recent past, as I desperately try to make sense of a world that feels out of balance.

As an AIDS activist, I marched in the streets for years, got arrested over and over again, screamed and yelled until I lost my voice and my faith in humanity. I was dejected, disillusioned, and grieving. It was my yoga practice that gave me a way back, that lifted me out of that hole. My practice has continued to be my main support over all these years, and I feel a debt of gratitude that I must find a way to repay. I hope to translate my experience into something useful for you. I've found solace in the teachings. They've helped me integrate my spiritual practice with the reality of the suffering and pain in my life and in the world around me.

As with my last book, this one was also inspired by death. This time it was the death of my mother three years ago, and the death of my father last year. Their passing has been a transformational experience that has once again led me back to the teachings. It has been a wake-up call, facing my mortality and the limited time I have here on earth and how I'm spending my time and energy.

My mother died a few months after my fiftieth birthday, which was a milestone that felt more like falling off a cliff. Her death made me feel disconnected, ungrounded, and basically lost. That was also the same year that my daughter's mental health challenges really came to a head. It was a rough time. I was diagnosed with an anxiety disorder, which has turned out to be one of my greatest teachers, but not one I would have chosen.

The years since have included COVID-19, my second pandemic, which has unearthed the trauma I experienced from AIDS. The struggle of these unusual times has inspired me to want to share my perspective on the yoga teachings, and the way I'm practicing and sharing them, in the hope that it's useful to you.

I've spent this time trying to learn how to mother myself, and how to be in the world in a different way. My thirty-year yoga practice was helpful, but it was not enough. I've had to learn to practice in a new way—a way that is not only healing for me as an individual but resonant with the suffering in the world around me. I've found that my healing lies not only in my personal practice, but in my connection with others. I've been reminded that taking care of myself was the first step in serving the world, and that is what spirituality is all about: service.

In addition to my practice, gardening has been one of my main tools for healing. The plants and trees live and die without anxiety. The earth embraces them as they go through their process of life and death. It supports their growth and recycles them as they die to give life to future generations. After all, soil, which is the foundation of life, is made of dead plants. I trust that my mind is a reflection of Mother Earth and that something new is growing from the soil of death and suffering I've experienced.

*Yoga Revolution* is a seed I'm planting in my own heart, and maybe in yours. It's about allowing for a full spectrum of possibilities—allowing for joy and sorrow to exist at the same time, and for all the states in between. It's radical acceptance combined with radical empathy. And that's what

I'll explore in this book: How do I take care of myself and serve the world without losing myself and also without making it all about me?

This is the way my mind works when my heart is open. It's a reaction against a limited view of the yoga practices that teach us to stop the thoughts in the mind. This is a literal interpretation of Patanjali's famous teaching *yogash chitta vritti nirodhah*, "stillness of the mind is yoga," which often leads to frustration in practitioners. Instead, it's time for a new interpretation. A revolutionary practice allows me to embrace the reality of my mind's creativity and electric spontaneity. Rather than fight my mind and tell it to, "Hush!" I'm celebrating its cleverness, humor, and complexity. My mind is such a useful tool. The question is whether I use it for my own selfish motives, or if I can find a way to be of service in the world. *Yoga Revolution* presents a new kind of mindfulness, a mind-full-ness!

To be honest, I get concerned with the endless talk of mindfulness without the embodied practices of yoga. To me, mindfulness is an advanced practice that comes from first working to get back into my body—and this is where yoga excels. Yoga offers a spectrum of practices to reinhabit my body, and eventually my mind. The yoga teachings are the key to cultivating this kind of open, loving space within me, which also reveals how deeply I'm connected to others.

Mindfulness is also not a panacea that removes the real harm that occurs in the world. We need to find a new way of approaching mindfulness and yoga that is engaged in service and social justice. Although, in the end, it's not really new. Yogic concepts were the root of Gandhi's revolution and the philosophies of Martin Luther King Jr. and Nelson Mandela. The yoga teachings are some of the most revolutionary in the world, and yet they have been commodified and capitalized into a neutral form of "whitewashed" exercise.

A yoga revolution is simply the reflection of a full heart in an open mind. This is a mind that accepts differences and rejects injustice and oppression. We usually think of the goal of yoga and meditation as an empty mind and a kind of self-absorbed transcendence. This concept is passed down from a monastic lineage that feels out of step with the path of the householder that most of us are walking. Our job is not to empty the mind, but to expand it so widely that it can embrace the entire universe.

Expanding the mind is simply allowing for creativity, intuition, and generosity. These last few years, my self-care also included a journey back into some of the pursuits I loved as a child, namely drawing. I see that creativity is embodied spirituality. Through creativity we connect to the energy of creation. Ironically, this is often lacking from spiritual practice. We are told how to practice without being given creative license to explore on our own. Even worse, we are often scolded for being undisciplined and disrespectful if we don't follow tradition.

There is a tension between making yoga accessible in creative ways and respecting the ancient lineages, culture, and traditions of yoga. With that in mind, we'll look at how to approach yoga practice in an original, and yet respectful, way. We'll discuss how to create a practice that can inspire and energize us with an eye for self-care and community care, which is service. We'll also get inspired by the way contemporary yoga activists are engaging with the practices through the contributions of some amazing guest teachers throughout the book.

*Yoga Revolution* is about tackling the challenge that Arjuna faces in the Bhagavad Gita: "Should I act?" It's about cultivating a state of mind that helps us figure out some of the hardest questions in life—when to speak up and when to step back. It's about creating space for us to hold opposing opinions, reconciling my own selfishness and yours.

This is the inner work that informs our actions in the world. Expanding our heart in our practice allows us to make choices based on love and compassion, which translates into positive change in the world. Generosity, kindness, and service all flow out of love. But to feel that love we need to do the necessary inner work of reflection, self-analysis, and discernment.

Before we go any further, I want to clarify a few things. I'm a yoga practitioner and teacher, and I don't pretend to be an authority on anything except for my own experience. I'm definitely not a scholar or historian, and I'm not enlightened (at least not any more than you are). My hope is that this book will be received in the way it is being offered—as a gentle nudge to bring a fresh perspective to the profound and transformative teachings of yoga to support ourselves as we change the world.

Throughout the book I quote selections from many different translations of Patanjali's Yoga Sutras and the Bhagavad Gita. I love exploring the different ways that masterful teachers and academics have interpreted these ancient texts, and I've chosen from many different versions in a completely subjective way. I hope these references inspire you to study these scriptures on your own and to find translations that speak to you.

These are the guiding lights of my practice, and I think all yoga practitioners can gain from getting to know these source texts and others. It's also important to revisit these texts at different times in our lives as we continually unearth our own unconscious biases. New interpretations often offer insights unavailable to earlier translators because of changes in cultural norms and understanding.

As we go along, I offer practice prompts. These are questions for you to reflect on. If you enjoy writing, spend a moment reflecting on these questions and then try journaling about them. If you don't enjoy writing, another option is to draw a picture or simply doodle (which is my favorite way to process information). Or you can sit and meditate on these questions by reading them and then closing your eyes and repeating them to yourself. Or even better, recline in a restorative yoga pose and ask yourself the question.

After you read it, listen for an answer. Rather than question yourself in a critical or analytical way, see if you can relax into an answer. Listening can mean opening your mind to an internal voice, or sometimes a fleeting image, that seemingly comes from nowhere. Try listening to yourself with compassion, the way you might listen to someone you love.

The book is organized into three parts. The first part is a reflection on the traditional teachings of yoga, and how you can approach them from where you are right now. I share a very personal interpretation of the teachings, offered with respect and love, but with an eye to the way the teachings speak to equity and justice and how they lead to compassion. The second part is a call to action—encouragement to integrate the teachings into the way you engage in the world. It includes ideas and encouragement for taking yoga off the mat, to have compassion for yourself and others, and to have the courage to speak up when you see harm happening in the world. The last part is about building a personal yoga practice that is authentic and supportive, to give you strength and courage as you move through your life.

These three parts reflect the need for us to constantly turn inward as we move out into the world. It's like a wave on the shore, reaching out into the world and then receding back into the ocean. A yoga revolution begins with our personal practice, grounded in the ancient teachings. The practices allow us to turn within to find truth, love, and compassion. Then with courage we reach back out into the world and serve.

# PART ONE

---

# INNER REVOLUTION

It must begin with you and me. All great things start on a small scale, all great movements begin with individuals; and if we wait for collective action, such action, if it takes place at all, is destructive and conducive to further misery. So revolution must begin with you and me.

—J. KRISHNAMURTI

# 1 | ANCIENT TEACHINGS, CONTEMPORARY PRACTICE

THE FIRST SECTION OF this book is an exploration of the essential yoga teachings in light of this current moment in time. I'm interested in looking back to the teachings and finding threads of service and social justice weaving their way through them. I don't think this is revisionist, or simply a matter of interpretation. I believe the teachings are showing us how to open our hearts and minds to see beyond our normally limited, self-centered vision of ourselves and the world. My vision of yoga is a unifying force, connecting us across time and space—even connecting us across the space that separates us by belief system and political affiliation.

## LIVING YOGA

Yoga is a revolutionary practice that changes our relationship with ourselves and with the world. First, consider the fact that yoga philosophy is completely at odds with contemporary capitalist culture. The basic concept of yoga is that we have what we need within, as opposed to the idea that we have to buy happiness or get happiness through external gratification.

Additionally, yoga has the ability to transform our relationship with our own mind—to cultivate an inner revolution. Yoga's ancient techniques offer guidance for cultivating a discerning, sensitive, and conscious inner life, which is what I'll discuss at length in this book. Yoga can make us compassionate and give us the courage to act on that compassion. This is a huge shift that can change the way we relate to other people, and it has major implications for our society at large. If the millions of people around the world who currently practice yoga could engage with this aspect of practice, we would see drastic changes in the world.

This is the first, most essential step in making change in the world and achieving social justice. Individual practitioners, you and me, engage with the practices in such a way that we no longer move from a place of us versus them. We no longer live only for ourselves, but in service to all humanity. I believe the evolution of humanity hinges on our ability to transcend our limited egocentric thinking, and to me this is the very essence of yoga: to think of the collective rather than simply ourselves. Amazingly, we may find that our own happiness and joy expand in direct correlation to the well-being of the collective. True wellness only exists in community, and that is what the teachings have been telling us all along. We just haven't been listening.

## HONORING THE YOGA TRADITION

Whenever we talk about yoga, we need to first stop and consider the essential yoga teachings and exactly what we are grounding our practice in. My training and study have been in the Yoga Sutras of Patanjali and the Bhagavad Gita. I realize there are a multitude of other ancient yoga scriptures, but since I've spent so much time with these two texts, this is where I always return for inspiration and guidance. I also feel strongly that we haven't yet applied the teachings from these texts to our contemporary yoga practice and to our lived experience. So I go back to them again and again, as I have for over thirty years.

It's important to note that these two texts offer divergent paths. Patanjali's path is one of renunciation designed for monks, while the Gita offers a path of service. I think it's time to integrate Patanjali's brilliant teachings on gaining mental clarity with a new focus on creating an engaged yoga. If, like me, you're living as a householder, that means you are engaging with society through relationships, through work, and through other aspects of an organized society. These social systems are guided by politics and the laws that firmly insert politics into our daily lives. If you're a householder yoga practitioner, then your practice demands an additional level of social awareness. You don't have to call it politics, but there is a way that your practice automatically becomes socially engaged because your life is. Practicing yoga is not an excuse to ignore what is happening around you. So, unless you're a monk, you really have no excuse.

Modern scholars question whether the Yoga Sutras, in particular, deserve the attention they receive. The history of yoga is complex and confusing, because there is not a single yoga to trace back over time (especially since it's such a long time). Instead we can find threads of themes shifting and growing according to culture and context. For example, the traditions that focus on *bhakti* yoga, the devotional practices, or *hatha* yoga, the physical practices.

In James Mallinson and Mark Singleton's landmark book, *Roots of Yoga*, which was just released a few years ago, we see a renewed attempt to reveal additional scriptural sources for information about the history of yoga. They also discuss the Yoga Sutras of Patanjali and its relationship to the other texts. "The influence of Buddhism is also evident in the text, and the *Patanjalayogashastra* represents a Brahmanical attempt to appropriate yoga from the Shramana traditions."[1] In other words, the Yoga Sutras, correctly referred to as the *Patanjalayogashastra*, may have been an attempt to formalize the ascetic yoga tradition (*shramana*) by the Brahmin, priestly, caste. This may also have contributed to later efforts by the colonizing British to control the culture of India, and it adds yet another dimension to the complex history of yoga.

My teacher, Swami Satchidananda, whom I'll talk more about later, was part of a monastic yoga lineage that goes back many generations. These days there doesn't seem to be much credence given to these traditional guru lineages because of all the harm that has been done in them. In fact, I don't think there is a single lineage that is free from an abuse scandal.

As we enter a time of post-lineage yoga, the question is whether the community itself can step forward to hold the teachings.[2] This is what I've seen happen in the global Accessible Yoga community, and in my own life. I see a community learning how to support itself. Personally, I feel grateful that I was part of a traditional lineage, even though I see clearly the dangers of such a structure. I don't think a lineage is essential for the transmission of the teachings, but we have to do a better job of sharing and supporting each other if the community is going to replace the guru.

It's helpful to consider that these teachings come from a different time and place—ancient South Asia. The teachings derive ideas from the earliest Indian texts, the Vedas, which are classed as *shruti*, meaning they were "heard" by visionary poets. "The Vedas are not thought to have been revealed to a certain person or persons at a specific historical moment; they are believed to have always existed and were apprehended by sages in deep meditative states at some point prior to c. 1500 B.C.E. but precisely when is unknown."[3]

There are many embodied spiritual traditions, similar to yoga, found in other indigenous cultures. In the end, what is clear is that yoga is a group of ancient indigenous practices and ideas that have a very long and complex history.[4] Political forces and commercial interests continue to shape our understanding of the practice, and it's important to consider the political or financial interests of any source you are studying.

These sacred teachings have been used, and even weaponized, for thousands of years in India and now across the world. For example, the caste system is a form of oppression that kept many Indians from accessing these teachings or even speaking Sanskrit.[5] Similarly, modern postural yoga has used a version of the teachings that exclude many people from the practice. The underlying question is whether we can find universal truth in both ancient and modern yoga and distill those truths into something that we can practice. Although yoga may not always have been taught or shared equitably, the essence of the teaching is true equality, and it is based on the idea that we all share the same essence.

Thankfully, these days there seems to be a renewed interest in sharing the true heart of yoga in the midst of a contemporary practice that feels sanitized and overly commercial. We're finally hearing directly from contemporary South Asian teachers, who offer an essential perspective on the teachings. Susanna Barkataki, in her book *Embrace Yoga's Roots: Courageous Ways to Deepen Your Yoga Practice*, offers a glimpse into how we can approach yoga today in a way that is respectful to the tradition, rather than culturally appropriating it.

By connecting these teachings to our contemporary lives and current challenges, we can show our respect and create a bridge from past to present. Yoga offers universal spiritual teachings, and it is our job to make the connection to this moment and this place. After sharing the ethical teachings of *yama* (abstentions) and *niyama* (observances), which we'll discuss in detail later, Patanjali explains: "These great vows are universal, not limited by class, place, time, or circumstance."[6] In essence, these are teachings for all people for all time. There's a powerful message there. Lessons that were

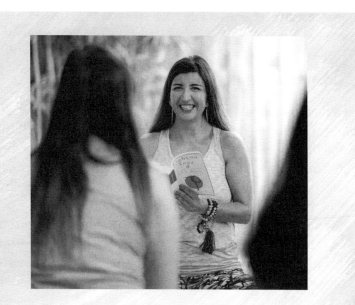

## SUSANNA BARKATAKI

As someone raised within the yoga tradition, there is no distinction between yoga, *seva*, and social justice. My *aita*, my paternal grand-mother from Assam, Lakshmi Devi Barkataki, served anyone who came by her doorstep. She embodied seva, which means "generous service."

Whatever leads us toward unity is yoga.

My *jethai*, my father's elder sister, embodies care and action in the face of injustice.

Whatever causes separation, within ourselves or with others, is not yoga.

Yoga is something that I learned how to be, not just do. Unity isn't some idealistic dream that we can just wish into being. Skipping over the often-divided reality we live within isn't the solution. Pretending separation and suffering don't exist is not the fastest way to unity.

This is why yoga naturally emerges in practice as a science of care, equity, and justice. I aim to address the causes of separation to practice yoga as unity.

shared from teacher to student thousands of years ago are still reaching us across the ocean of time.

## UNIVERSAL AND TIMELESS TEACHINGS

I just want to pause and say that it feels almost impossible to comprehend such a vast amount of time. My mind seems to understand the idea of the past and the future, and the concept of a distant past is comprehensible, but it's hard to differentiate between something a few hundred years old and something a few thousand years old. I get stuck on the thought of yoga teachings existing for 3,500 years or more.

It's so interesting how time seems to rush or stop throughout our lives. One minute of waiting can feel like forever, yet a lifetime flashes before our eyes. And I swear, as I get older, time seems to flow even faster. In fact, according to recent research, the experience of time actually does speed up as we get older.[7]

While the teachings are timeless and universal, our circumstances have changed. We have no choice but to interpret the teachings and apply them to this moment. In fact, that is what these ancient scriptures ask us to do: *Atha yoga anushasanam*, "Now, further instruction on yoga."[8] We are always being asked to take one step further—to dive deep into the meaning of the texts, rather than to float on the surface of the words.

Those surface interpretations can become a way of keeping the power of the teachings exclusive, rather than making them accessible and useful. According to the Bhagavad Gita, "In flowery discourses, the unwise focus on the letter of scripture and say there is nothing else."[9] Fundamentalism exists in all religions and spiritual traditions, and we need to be aware of it and the way it functions. Focusing on the letter of scripture and saying there is nothing else is a way to limit our access to the power of these teachings. On the other hand, making the practices widely available and accessible, especially to marginalized groups, is an essential aspect of living yoga authentically. To do so, we need to earnestly study the teachings, uncover their essence, and find ways to apply them to our lives right now.

Of course, we need to be aware of our own prior conditioning and the way we have been trained to think and to see the world. Our experience of these ancient teachings is tinted by the culture we live in right now. So how do we find the truth, or the true meaning? First, we need to become aware of our own personal biases and "positionality," the social and political context that supports our identity.[10] That means reflecting on our proximity to power and the ways we have experienced prejudice and oppression, or not. This isn't about assigning blame, rather it's an essential part of our practice because our personal background and experiences distort our vision of the world.

> Explore your implicit biases by completing a free online implicit association test. Harvard University has a variety of tests that look at issues of race, gender, disability, and so on.[11]

For something to be universal and timeless it must ring true in our hearts. So I would suggest you find your own way in by studying multiple translations and interpretations of the ancient scriptures. In this book, I'm relying on many different teachers and authors for translations because I don't think there is just one way to understand or interpret these teachings. I'm simply sharing what is most meaningful to me. Personally, my process is to study different translations and then ask myself, "Does what I'm reading connect to my own intuitive wisdom and intersect with my understanding of yoga so far?"

When you've read a few different translations you can begin to get a sense of where they overlap and where they are different. You can also begin to see different translators' perspectives. It's very helpful when they offer the Sanskrit words as well so you can study them directly. Although I realize this is a more controversial statement than it sounds like because, traditionally, only certain castes were allowed to read Sanskrit.

Studying these scriptures directly is a practice of *svadhyaya*, a term that Patanjali uses to describe this process of study. Actually, the word *svadhyaya* can be interpreted as study of the self as well as study of the Vedas. If you think about it, they are really one and the same. When we look deep within ourselves we find the truth in our heart. That same truth is found in all the world's ancient faith traditions. How could it be otherwise? Studying the Vedas, and the scriptures that flowed from them, we can find ourselves. This process is different than simply reading a book. We find truth in a scripture, and then pause and look into our own heart to find that truth reflected there.

The next step is to ask yourself, "Is my practice useful?" The true test of the universality of the teachings is how well we can implement them in our lives right now, literally thousands of years after they were first shared. That is one of the goals of this book, answering the question, "Can I live yoga now?" Personally, I'm not a historian. I know that many people are doing that academic work, which is wonderful. I'm a yoga practitioner, and what I'm searching for is an understanding of these traditional teachings to apply to my life. I don't just want to study yoga. I want to live yoga. That is why this is a completely subjective book based on my experience and what I've found in my practice.

I hope to share what I've found with you, as well as suggest how you can apply this wisdom in your life. That's a big part of this project, and my work in general, over the past twenty-five years trying to make yoga accessible. I want to support you in cultivating a useful and effective yoga practice that works for you right now and also serves the collective.

One of the biggest misunderstandings that I've faced over the course of my teaching career is the idea that I'm trying to make yoga accessible by adapting or modifying the practices. That has never been my goal. I'm not interested in changing yoga into something else. What I have tried to do is to excavate the truth of the teachings, and find the truths that are already universal, meaning that they apply to all of us no matter our ability or background. Also, my interest is in taking what often seem like esoteric and confusing ideas and trying to make them more easily understood—more accessible. In that way, this book is a continuation of my first book, *Accessible Yoga*, which mostly focused on making yoga asana available to anyone who is interested in practicing.

> What does yoga mean to you? Reflect on what you've been told yoga means, and how you've actually experienced it in your life. Is there a difference between what you've been taught and what you've experienced?

## LIFE, LIBERTY, AND THE PURSUIT OF HAPPINESS

The liberation that yoga offers is both personal and communal. Personal liberation for me is freedom from my own patriarchal, capitalist thinking.

It's a freedom that allows me to be awake to the insidious ways I have internalized white supremacy. It's about cultivating an internal voice that is not constantly negative and putting myself down. It's an internal reckoning—an internal speaking truth to power.

A yoga revolution is experienced through our unshakable support of social justice that comes from the realization that we all share the same heart. But saying, "We're all one" is only true if everyone is given the same access to resources, and above all, access to justice and power. After all, that's the meaning of social justice—everyone in society has justice. That means we are all treated fairly and equally. Unfortunately, marginalized people don't have equal access to power, and therefore we are not all one, at least not yet.

The basic idea is that the U.S. Declaration of Independence was actually speaking the truth when it declared "We hold these truths to be self-evident, that all men [sic] are created equal, that they are endowed by their Creator with certain unalienable Rights, that among these are Life, Liberty and the pursuit of Happiness." Our personal liberation and that of our community are not separate things.

It's not all love and light. It's about admitting that there are ongoing police killings born from systemic racism, and that my selfishness has contributed to this situation because I've told myself I'm too busy to do anything about it. It's the truth of a climate disaster my children will inherit, and the fact that we act like it's not happening.

Instead, let's ask ourselves how we can make real change in the world. Let's allow our practice to inspire us to create, to question, and to act. Can your practice get your mind clear enough to find space and time to engage in politics: to vote, call your representatives, do some community service, or even run for office?

I realize this is a departure from Patanjali's focus on quieting the mind so that we can detach from the world and transcend it completely. But we need to be more clear about who these teachings were designed for, and contrast that with our lives today. In contemporary yoga we still hear the echo of a monastic desire to leave society, and it sounds a lot like spiritual bypass. That's the conscious, or unconscious, desire to avoid the painful parts of life. You have to admit, it is deeply ironic that we've taken the asceticism of our monastic past and mixed it with enough New Age gobbledygook to transform it into a path that we expect to be lined only in love and light, a path so focused on our individuality that we have lost our humanity. So the question that we're left with is this: How do we cultivate an engaged yoga practice that is both respectful to its ancient roots and yet responsive to the reality of our sometimes confusing and often painful lives today?

White supremacy and systemic racism have poisoned the water to the point that our personal practice alone can't make it drinkable. But, our practice can give us the clarity to step up to the task of making real political and social change. The focus of this book is the inner work that each of us faces as we pursue a spiritual practice. For the political work, it's important to listen to the leaders in the community who understand what action needs to be taken. I'm just trying to encourage and support the essential internal part of the process.

## TOWARD A QUEER YOGA

We each have a different role to play in creating an equitable and just world. The challenge is getting clear about our role and standing shoulder to shoulder with others who are doing their own work. We are working separately, but together, toward liberation. This brings to mind the image of the rainbow, the symbol of the queer community, which I feel so blessed to be a part of. Our community is constantly teaching the world how to embrace differences, how to love, and how to be human on a spectrum of gender. My personal struggles as a cisgender queer white middle-aged Jewish man have been mild compared to what so many queer people endure for living their truth. Some are emotionally and physically tortured and even killed.

Gay sex was illegal in the United States when I came out of the closet in 1984 and, shockingly, it's still illegal in many countries and punishable by death in eleven countries.[12] In the United States, there are major inequities within the queer community. In particular, trans women of color have an incredibly high murder rate that goes mostly unnoticed and unchecked by society.[13] Black trans women started the modern gay rights movement and are often on the cutting edge of social change, yet they don't often benefit from these movements because of systemic racism and transphobia.[14] The Stonewall riots, which were the spark that led to the modern gay rights movement, were led by Marsha P. Johnson and other trans women of color.[15]

Stonewall is a good example of rioting, and protest in general, as a force for positive change. The queer community had been oppressed for so long and denied basic human rights. Stonewall was an opportunity to speak up against an oppressive system that kept us as not only second-class citizens, but complete outcasts. Similarly, I've seen some confusion within the yoga community about the ethics of protesting during the Black Lives Matter movement, and I think the issue is one of basic human rights. If the system that you're living in doesn't respect your basic human rights, then protesting that system is ethical. In other words, supporting oppressive systems is unethical, and it's our job as yoga practitioners to speak up against suffering wherever we see it. That's the heart of *ahimsa*, non-harm.

I bow to the queer leaders who are out there on the edge being themselves and challenging norms. I bow to our siblings lost to AIDS and celebrate the fact that as outsiders we can shine a bright beam of light on culture in a way that forces all of us to not look away. Although I feel protective of the queer community, I also know there is so much that we can teach the world. A queer sensibility is so often at the forefront of cultural transformation and renewal. The renewal I'm seeking is an embodied spirituality that catalyzes concrete change. I pray that this book helps lead to a small shift in our shared consciousness toward a place of acceptance, openness, and positive action.

I'm hoping to share the gift of the challenges I've faced. My experience as a queer person has made me stronger and more capable of love and compassion—because I know what it's like to *not* be loved and to *not* receive compassion. This is the hidden power of the oppressed: the ability to free ourselves and others. We've seen this time and time again throughout history: Black trans women leading the gay rights movement, Black people showing us what justice actually looks like through Black Lives Matter. According to Paulo Freire, in his groundbreaking work, *Pedagogy of the Oppressed*:

> This, then, is the great humanistic and historical task of the oppressed: to liberate themselves and their oppressors as well. The oppressors, who oppress, exploit, and rape by virtue of their power, cannot find in this power the strength to liberate either the oppressed or themselves. Only power that springs from the weakness of the oppressed will be sufficiently strong to free both.[16]

With this I mind, I hope to highlight the gifts of our shared suffering and consider how we can use that suffering to free ourselves and others. With this possibility in mind, I shine a light on the Yoga Sutras of Patanjali, but this isn't Mr. Iyengar's light on the Sutras. This is a queer rainbow of sparkling light shining from the twenty-first century. What I see in the Sutras is a pathway for personal liberation that emphasizes a loving, engaged, and extremely discerning mind. This is different from the traditional story we hear in the Sutras that feels more like the sad tale of a lonely soul searching for its own absolution.

I also bow to the wisdom of the Bhagavad Gita, the song of God, and listen to the story of Arjuna, a person torn apart by the challenges of life. The Gita shows us how to transform our contemplative practice into action through service—action born from love. Krishna teaches us how our practice makes the mind clear so that we know how to act for the highest good. This is what the Gita calls "skill in action," the ultimate goal of yoga. This is also the title of the groundbreaking book by Michelle Cassandra Johnson, who approaches the idea of applying these ancient teachings to address the contemporary issue of racism and white supremacy.

## NONATTACHMENT IS PURE LOVE

The yoga teachings were designed for male monastics thousands of years ago, so it makes sense that we've had to translate them and interpret them to apply to our twenty-first-century householder lifestyle. But why have we stood by and allowed yoga to be cherry-picked for the ideas that reinforce a modern, self-centered approach to life? Unfortunately, many of the most popular teachers, and sources of the teachings, have been equally self-centered and self-aggrandizing. It's really not surprising that the way we've come to understand yoga is based on the people who've popularized it.

This rather small group of yoga influencers includes some very abusive and greedy individuals. For example, the famous Bikram Choudhury, who was selling yoga and Rolls-Royces to the rich and famous as he cheated and abused his students.[17] Additionally, we have corporate interests that have appropriated yoga teachings into a lifestyle they could sell back to us. The essence of yoga can't be purchased, but that's not what we've been told. In the end, it's really no wonder we're confused.

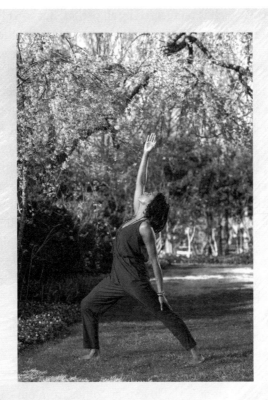

## MICHELLE CASSANDRA JOHNSON

I do not see my practice of yoga as separate from the work I do to create a just world. They are one and the same to me. The way I practice and what I choose to center as the practice of yoga are focused on how we create a just world. Yoga is about selfless service, devotion, and knowledge. These paths are important keys to us realizing a world in which we all can be free. My practice of meditation and movement as well as the study of the Bhagavad Gita provide emotional and spiritual sustenance to me. This nourishment from spiritual practice allows me to fully see with clarity the ways in which injustice persists on our planet. Being spiritually fed pushes me to strive to do everything I do in my practice off of my cushion or mat in service to the collective good and our liberation.

Luckily, yoga itself is unaffected by all of that. But what is impacted is our connection to the teachings and the way we perceive them. A perfect example of a teaching that has been misunderstood is the essential concept of nonattachment, *vairagya*, which is freedom from selfish desire. Traditionally, nonattachment was understood to mean not having personal relationships and belongings. Monks were taught to not have personal relationships so they could cultivate a relationship with God. But as householders, thousands of years later, we have to find a new way to relate to this idea that is literally the bedrock that yoga philosophy is built on.

Rather than focusing on what nonattachment is asking us to give up, we can focus on what it's teaching us to reach for. For contemporary householder practitioners, nonattachment is not about renouncing all our relationships so we can find God. It's about finding God in our relationships—seeing God in others. This is an essential difference between Patanjali's message and the message of the Gita, even though both texts are asking us to practice nonattachment.

To put it simply, nonattachment is asking us to get over ourselves, and to truly embrace others as if our very survival depends on it—our survival, not only as individuals, but as a planet. Sometimes confusion arises in spiritual practice because attachment and nonattachment both stem from love. It's just that attachment is the love that comes from our ego-mind, and nonattachment is the love that flows from our heart. Nonattachment is pure, selfless love. This is the highest form of spirituality: a compassion so wide that it includes the entire universe in its wake.

It's also worth noting that as social justice activists, we need to be non-attached to the outcome of our work. Cultural shifts can be slow, and we don't always see the results of our efforts right away. Patience with the work and with ourselves is essential so that we can keep up our energy and stay focused over a long arc of time.

## YOGA BEGINS WITH BEING KIND TO YOURSELF

I want to mention an important point about noticing the quality of your thoughts as you read this book, and really anytime you are engaging in mindfulness or yoga. Simply put, be kind to yourself. Have compassion for yourself. Try not to use these teachings as a way to condemn yourself.

Rather, focus on what you can do, how you can move forward, and how you can make productive change.

Most spiritual books, and many teachers, use our weaknesses against us. We're asked to move from a place of deficit and need, as if we're completely ignorant. I want to suggest another way: Can you come to these reflections with your best self? Can you begin yoga already full from what life has taught you and from an inner knowing? According to these teachings, the truth already lies inside our heart, so none of this is really new to us. It's just a matter of remembering something you may have forgotten or put aside.

Yoga is remembering what you've forgotten—the truth lies within you. It's like Dorothy in the *Wizard of Oz* (a story that may actually have been influenced by yoga philosophy[18]), when she is told at the end of the story that she's had the answer in her possession all along. After seeking the advice of Oz himself, and realizing there's no one behind the curtain, Dorothy pleads with Glinda the Good Witch, "Oh, will you help me? Can you help me?" Glinda finally explains to Dorothy, "You don't need to be helped any longer. You've always had the power. . . ."

I find that the most thoughtful, caring, and sensitive people seem to be the hardest on themselves. I guess it's understandable that the qualities of introspection and inquisitiveness go along with self-doubt and self-criticism. It's unfortunate, because these qualities are incredibly powerful and, I would add even essential, for successful spiritual practice. Hardheadedness is not conducive to spiritual awakening—kindness is. And that includes kindness to yourself.

I realize that it's easier said than done, and I know from personal experience that sensitive people tend to use spiritual teachings to beat themselves up. We look at the teachings, and instead of seeing a path forward, all we see is how far away we are from our goal. Why is it that when we identify a goal, all we see is the distance to that goal, instead of appreciating the fact that we have found a clear path?

Just this morning, I got a message from a longtime student telling me she was struggling emotionally. She said she was having a lot of family issues, and she was very upset about it. Mostly she was struggling with her aging parents. At the end of her message she added a point that got my attention. She said, in a self-deprecating way, "I see how emotional I am and how many attachments I have!" As if she was a failure as a yoga practitioner for loving her parents!

Remember, the teaching of nonattachment is meant to be an empowering message of independence and pure love. Nonattachment represents the fullness of our spiritual being, unaffected by the world. But, as with so many things in life, we have used the teachings to be hard on ourselves, to criticize, and to put ourselves down. Our attachment to others reflects our ability to love another person, and it is literally the definition of our humanity. Why would we want to deny that?

If the goal truly is letting go of our attachments, the first step is to forgive ourselves for having them in the first place. Forgiveness releases us from self-criticism and allows us to see our actions, as well as other people's actions, more clearly. Once we've forgiven ourselves for being human, we can truly embody our humanity. Then we can forgive others and release ourselves from our attachments to their behavior.

I thought it might be helpful for my student to consider her ability to love her family, and the immense capacity for love that her pain represents, as a gift. So, I responded to her by saying, "Attachments are actually very beautiful. At least they make us human." My challenge for her, and for all of us, is this: Instead of criticizing yourself for being loving, could you celebrate your capacity for love and the courage you have to expose your broken heart to the world over and over again?

To me, this is the fragile power of a yoga practitioner. We don't hide away from the world to protect ourselves from pain, instead we dive in headfirst, with heart open. We are courageous. We know we will experience pain, but we love anyway without abandon, and hopefully, without attachment.

Unfortunately, putting ourselves down and constantly diminishing our abilities can lead to confusion, rather than to realization. As with everything in life, we need to find balance—the middle path. It's important to clearly see the impact our attachments have on our mind and the way we interpret the world. Our minds are literally colored by our beliefs and desires, and our experiences are being filtered through those beliefs.

It reminds me of the concept of "confirmation bias," which is defined by the American Psychological Association as, "the tendency to gather evidence that confirms preexisting expectations, typically by emphasizing or pursuing supporting evidence while dismissing or failing to seek contradictory evidence."[19] To me, the revolution of yoga lies in our ability to question our biases and to analyze our limitations in the context of a well-defined practice.

This calm self-analysis takes a lot of inner strength and conviction, but most importantly, it takes a firm grounding in yoga itself. The point isn't to throw all your beliefs in the trash and beat yourself up for not being a good yoga practitioner. Rather, it's about analyzing the mind and exploring your heart in the context of the yoga teachings, which can provide us that special balance of strength and love that is courage and compassion.

Similarly, when you open a new yoga book, take a new yoga class, or attend a new training, you don't need to throw away everything you know and start again. Instead, be discriminating and consider all that you're learning in context. Carefully consider new ideas and practices. Ruminate on them and check in with how they feel to you. If they seem true and useful, then digest them; if not, spit them out. Trust your intuition and allow your study and practice to refine your understanding and give form to what you know in your heart.

This approach to yoga practice takes tremendous courage to begin, but thankfully, offers us more courage in exchange. That's the courage to embrace yourself in all your glory and in all your failures, and the compassion to embrace others in the same way. Personally, I no longer aspire to a transcendental yogic experience outside of society, isolated, or beyond this reality. I aspire to an embodied practice of justice in action that acknowledges that my liberation is not only bound up in yours, but is the same as yours. An inner revolution begins with an open mind prepared to love and serve in the name of equity and justice.

Can you think of an attachment that you have to someone in your life? What happens if you let go of what you need from that person and focus on the love you feel for them instead?

## 2 | THE GOAL OF YOGA: CLEAR PERCEPTION

A Dialectic—Seemingly Opposing Truths
*di·a·lec·tic*
1. the art of investigating or discussing the truth of opinions.
2. inquiry into metaphysical contradictions and their solutions.[1]

WHY DOES IT ALWAYS seem like truth is found inside a paradox? Can two seemingly opposing ideas both be true? When we start examining big questions, the answers almost always include some kind of contradiction, or dialectic. For me, one of the most important practices of yoga has been consciously opening to different ways of thinking. I try to allow for contradictions to exist in my mind—giving both ideas space to breathe and exist. There is so often a dialectic—two seemingly opposing truths—in the teachings: We're the same, but we're different. Our time on earth is limited, but our spirit is immortal.

The ability to make space for this understanding is reflected in the way we think and speak. We often default to an "either/or" mindset rather than a "both/and" way of thinking. We want everything to be cut and dried, without allowing for the murky space of the unknown to exist. Can we allow for two emotions or contradictory thoughts to exist at the same time? "I love you, and I'm angry at you." "I'm anxious and excited." "My body is mortal, but my spirit is immortal."

It's like there are two sets of rules in life. The rules of the natural world and the rules of the spiritual world. One set of rules follows natural law: up and down, birth and death, hot and cold. That is the level of duality that exists in daily life. The other set of rules applies to a subtler aspect of experience, based in spirit.

In spiritual reality, we sense with our intuitive awareness. We notice that our hair stands on end before something bad happens, or we think of someone right before they call us. The way we experience the spiritual realm in daily life is often through emotion instead of thought. It's the sense that we are loved and connected to those we love. It's the knowledge that our ancestors are still here watching, loving, and guiding us, even though logically it doesn't make sense. It's the feeling that when someone dies, they are still present in our lives.

This spiritual reality is the space of feeling, existing, and being. It's the part of us that feels connected to others and to all of creation. Some call this God, or spirit. It's the part of me that is connected to you. It's my essence, the part of me that hasn't changed over the course of my entire life, while my body and mind constantly change. It's like spiritual gravity—the force that pulls all of us together. Remember, gravity doesn't just pull us toward the earth, it pulls any two masses together. And that's the nature of spirit, an interconnected network of being that is invisibly pulling us closer. We don't see gravity but we can feel it. Does that make it any less real?

> Think of your earliest memory, and connect to what was the same about you then and now. Was there a certain sense of self, or an awareness that hasn't changed over all this time when everything else seems to have changed?

## WHO AM I?

One of my earliest memories is of red tile floors—I was probably crawling on them. I also remember those tiles leading me to a green and white room where my grandmother was standing on her head. That image is stuck in my mind, and I wonder why. Is it because it was so unusual to see someone standing on her head, or is it because I had some sense that it was connected to yoga and to what I would spend my life pursuing?

Another early memory is of my grandmother teaching me to meditate, and my first thought was, "Oh yeah, I get this." It was as if I had meditated before. In that moment, I was connected to my intuitive awareness, to my spirit. Is that what you call a memory of the future, a premonition? There have been so many moments in life that have that same quality—a sense of knowing. Sometimes it was knowing that something was wrong, and sometimes it was knowing that something was right. There's no better feeling, knowing you're in the right place and moving in the right direction. Sometimes it's as simple as asking the right question.

> What is It that we worship as this Self? Which of the two is the Self? Is It that by which one sees, or that by which one hears, or that by which one smells odour, or that by which one utters speech, or that by which one tastes the sweet or the sour?
>
> It is this heart (intellect) and this mind that were stated earlier. It is sentience, rulership, secular knowledge, presence of mind, retentiveness, sense perception, fortitude, thinking, genius, mental suffering, memory, ascertainment resolution, life activities, hankering, passion and such others? All these verily are the names of Consciousness.[2]

This passage from the *Aitareya Upanishad* shows that we've been asking these same questions for eons. Which part of me is spirit and which part of me is mind? Sometimes these deep questions can leave us feeling hopeless, but often they have the opposite effect. Asking myself "who am I?" can give my heart a moment to step forward from behind the veil of the busy mind. I truly believe that if there is a force that animates me and all of creation, the more I can connect with and trust that force, the more I will be at peace with my mind and my life. The challenge is that I forget to trust. I get caught up in the duality.

## IDENTITY POLITICS

This same challenge of navigating duality applies to contemporary identity politics. On the one hand, I'm not interested in glorifying the suffering I've experienced as a queer person. But I also feel proud of myself for overcoming the challenges of being queer in a straight world. There is tremendous benefit in the growth that comes from struggling, but I also feel confident that I could be as strong and creative without the pain, maybe even stronger and more creative!

Logo of the Human Rights Campaign[3]

The paradox is that the struggle makes us grow, but at some point it will also stop our growth and literally kill us. We can see a clear example of this in the AIDS epidemic and in the way the queer community came together in a show of unity that revolutionized gay rights. But how many people died in the process? Actually, about 32.7 million people have died of AIDS around the world since the start of the epidemic.[4] That's too big a price to pay for improved rights for the living.

Another paradox is the way that marginalized folks are perceived by mainstream culture. We tend to be either idolized or vilified. This is yet another way that we avoid giving people basic human rights, by not seeing each other as simply human, as equals. The logo of the Human Rights Campaign is literally an equal sign. The HRC "envisions a world where every member of the LGBTQ family has the freedom to live their truth without fear, and with equality under the law." Queer and trans people are literally seeking equal rights, not special rights. Although many of us would like to go one step further and not simply fight for equality under the law, but reimagine a new legal, political, and cultural structure that emphasizes shared power and shared resources.

I know many people with disabilities who share that same feeling: pride for being disabled, but no interest in being put on a pedestal as "inspiration porn." Reclaiming the word *disabled* is an example of pride. Rather than put up with euphemisms for disability like *differently-abled*, the disability movement is taking back its power.

It's incredible to me that pioneers in the disability rights movement aren't household names. These are people who have led the charge for basic human rights for the largest minority group in the world—over one billion people around the world identify as part of this community. People like Ed Roberts, Judith Heumann, Ady Barkan, and Haben Girma are leaders whose stories we should learn about in school.

Still, the question remains: How do we move away from forcing marginalized people to excel in order to be treated with respect and receive equal rights? Privately, we need to ask ourselves when we can rest if we are constantly striving for that extra level of approval? I think the answer lies in the paradox: difference makes us stronger, but it also weakens us. We can have pride in our differences but still expect equal rights, equal treatment, and equal justice—not because we're the same as everyone but because we are equally deserving. We are human.

There's a similar paradox in the way individual social justice movements have ignored the intersectionality of their work: pitting us against each other. According to Kimberlé Crenshaw, who coined the phrase, "Intersectionality is a lens through which you can see where power comes and collides, where it interlocks and intersects. It's not simply that there's a race problem here, a gender problem here, and a class or LBGTQ problem there. Many times that framework erases what happens to people who are subject to all of these things."[5]

Intersectionality shows us the complexity of our identities and the ways they are interwoven. For example, we see racism in the queer community and homophobia in communities of color. We all have multiple aspects to our identity: ways that we have power and ways that we are powerless.

Yoga offers a way for us to clearly see our own oppression and the way we may be oppressing others. The teachings show us that we are all prejudiced in some way or another. It's the nature of the mind. Our experience of the world is tinted by our belief system, and the world we see is a reflection of our own mind. Yoga is a practice of cleaning our lens to experience the world in a more objective way. This begins with self-analysis and reflection, and it leads to compassion. By cultivating compassion for anyone who is suffering, we can see that other people are also oppressed and that we may be participating in that oppression in some way.

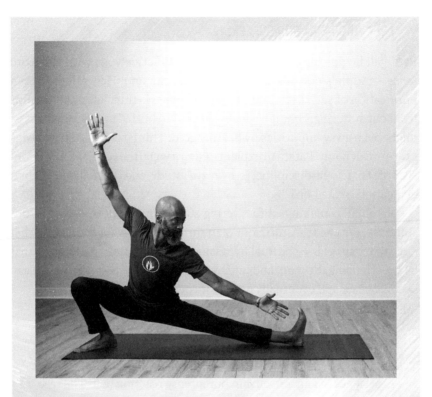

## YOGI J MILES

My service and social justice work has become my practice. I feel like I have lost the distinction between what it means to have a "yoga" practice and what it means to simply live my life according to my highest principles. Living in this Black body has never been so important as it seems to be now, and it feels nearly as dangerous as it has ever been. Being steeped in a practice that provides me with the tools to address my spirituality has also given me the tools to fully address my humanity. Yoga has given me the ability to address and attend to my own individual healing, and therefore my own personal liberation. There's safety within myself that no one can take away from me. I guess you could say that my yoga practice has given me courage.

## LEARNING FROM OUR SUFFERING

Patanjali begins his discussion on how to practice yoga with the word *tapas*—and he's not talking about Spanish cuisine! He's talking about purification or self-discipline. Sometimes *tapas* is translated as "learning from our suffering," but it basically means "to burn," in the way that you might burn away impurities by heating gold. This is why I often call yoga a form of alchemy. Patanjali explains, "*Kriya* yoga, the path of action, consists of (*tapas*) self-discipline, (*svadhyaya*) study, and (*ishvarapranidhana*) dedication to the Lord."[6]

Patanjali is making a life-altering statement about the value of our suffering. We can transform our pain through the alchemy of yoga. That doesn't mean we use spiritual bypassing to avoid suffering. It means that by experiencing the pain, and understanding why we're suffering, we can become wiser and eventually have more peace.

> There is great violence when we avoid our pain, because we become trapped in reacting to it as we target others as the reason for our hurt. This is why our anger and rage are dangerous. It is not the experience of anger itself, but our intense reaction to it. The reaction is also the avoidance of experiencing the experience of anger.
>
> —LAMA ROD OWENS[7]

I think this is one of the most misunderstood aspects of the yoga path. It is a path through suffering, not around it. Yoga practice begins with a willingness to learn from our pain and suffering—to feel it. The yoga begins when you lie on your mat and cry, not when you're doing some fancy pose. Or yoga begins when your partner says something that hurts your feelings, and you pause before snapping back with something hurtful in return.

I can give you an example. The other day, my husband made a comment about how when I water the plants on our porch, I'm not careful and the water gets all over the place. I remember noticing how quickly my mind started to think of a response—searching for something I could criticize him for. Then I paused and noticed what I was feeling. It was the pang of even this slight criticism. And this is the tricky part. Tapas isn't an invitation to accept abuse. It's increasing self-knowledge by shining a light on our unhealed trauma.

I still snapped back at my husband about how he doesn't water the plants at all. But, at least I saw my mind in action. I became more sensitive to the fact that when I'm in pain I don't respond in ways that are in alignment with my larger goals in life. For example, I love my husband and want to create a loving and supportive relationship with him. So, rather than snapping back, I could have shared honestly and said, "When you criticize me it hurts my feelings." The truth would have allowed him to get closer to me, rather than pushing him away by criticizing him in return.

The work of tapas is uncovering the reasons why I don't allow for greater intimacy in my life. This means understanding why I don't think I'm worthy of love. It includes lots of other incorrect beliefs, based on past traumas, that keep my mind in a reactive state. Tapas is the willingness to experience the suffering that comes my way rather than avoid pain through some addictive behavior or by blaming others.

I repeat, tapas is *not* an excuse to accept abuse. This point is especially important for anyone who has been abused, marginalized, or experienced trauma. Don't let spiritual practice become an excuse to accept abuse or allow yourself to be controlled by someone else, such as a teacher or guru. It's a skillful balancing act. How do we use our yoga practice to open our hearts and learn from our suffering, while not accepting abuse or avoiding pain through spiritual bypassing? Martin Luther King Jr. explained it so clearly when he said, "As my sufferings mounted I soon realized that there were two ways in which I could respond to my situation—either to react with bitterness or seek to transform the suffering into a creative force. I decided to follow the latter course."

Ultimately, I think it all works together in a beautiful choreography. Tapas is a gateway to empowerment. It's a way to transform our suffering and shift away from being a victim. But this is an internal process. We can transmute our suffering through these embodied practices. We experience anger, pain, frustration, disappointment, and grief in our body. So we need a physical and energetic practice like yoga to support the healthy processing of these emotions. This is a very personal experience, and it's not something we can tell someone else to do. In fact, I hesitate to even write about it because it can be so easily misunderstood and lead so quickly to victim blaming.

A classic example of tapas, and yoga in action, can be found in Viktor Frankl's classic work, *Man's Search for Meaning*. In this book, Frankl details his personal experience as a prisoner in a Nazi concentration camp, and he focuses on the ways that different prisoners responded to the suffering they experienced. Based on his experiences and observations, Frankl created a new approach to psychology focused on the idea that the ultimate need for humans is finding meaning in our lives and in our suffering.

> The way in which a man accepts his fate and all the suffering it entails, the way in which he takes up his cross, gives him ample opportunity—even under the most difficult circumstances—to add a deeper meaning to his life. It may remain brave, dignified and unselfish. Or in the bitter fight for self-preservation he may forget his human dignity and become no more than an animal. Here lies the chance for a man either to make use of or to forgo the opportunities of attaining the moral values that a difficult situation may afford him. And this decides whether he is worthy of his sufferings or not.
>
> Do not think that these considerations are unworldly and too far removed from real life. It is true that only a few people are capable of reaching such high moral standards. Of the prisoners only a few kept their full inner liberty and obtained those values which their suffering afforded, but even one such example is sufficient proof that man's inner strength may raise him above his outward fate. Such men are not only in concentration camps. Everywhere man is confronted with fate, with the chance of achieving something through his own suffering.[8]

## SPIRITUAL IGNORANCE

Frankl beautifully expresses the opportunities that arise from being "worthy of our suffering" and the concept of tapas. But, to me, there is another question here: How did we get to a point where Nazi concentration camps even existed? Shouldn't our response be outrage and political action? Is it enough to simply learn from our suffering and become masters of our own minds? Don't we also need to use our energy to create a world where there is less suffering for others, and where concentrations camps aren't a reality?

So there are two issues here: the way we respond to our own suffering and the way we respond to the suffering we see in others. These are two separate things, but they are intimately connected. The way I respond to my own suffering informs the way I respond to yours. Even though my suffering is an opportunity for my personal growth, it is in no way an excuse for others to allow that suffering to continue.

Similarly, when I see suffering in the world, it is my spiritual practice to have courageous compassion and act to reduce that suffering. I need both the courage to respond to my personal challenges with strength and the courage to speak up and act when I see harm occurring in the world. These two forms of courage are intimately connected: my inner practice dictates my outer actions.

The Yoga Sutras teach us that pain comes from having a limited vision of ourselves. We're stuck in the natural world, and we don't seem to have the ability to see beyond the body-mind to understand our spiritual nature. In sutra 2.15, Patanjali refers to this as ignorance, *avidya*, and goes as far as saying that *all* experiences in life are painful if we are completely identified with the body-mind.

> For one who has discrimination, everything is suffering on account of the suffering produced by the consequences [of action], by pain [itself], and by the *samskaras*, as well as on account of the suffering ensuing from the turmoil of the *vrittis* due to the *gunas*.⁹

In other words, we're screwed! Well, not really. What Patanjali is actually doing here so skillfully is frame his discussion in a positive way. Even though it may not seem that way at first. He starts with the assumption that we are spiritual beings (*purusha*) and we're having a temporary human experience (*prakriti*). Based on that vision of our lives it makes sense that any time we wrongly identify with the body-mind we experience pain. It's only when we are aligned with the truth of our existence, our spirit, that we're free from suffering.

Edwin Bryant, in his masterful translation of the Yoga Sutras of Patanjali, notes of sutra 2.15:

> This sutra is actually the pivot of this chapter, which, in turn, is the heart of the entire text. . . . The chapter thus echoes the Four

Noble Truths. One might ask, without an experience of the world as frustrating on some level, what would motivate one to seek fulfillment elsewhere and take up the rigors and challenges of the yoga path? If one perceives the world of experience as a jolly fine place in which to be, why would one wish to seek a higher truth? From this perspective, a recognition of the world as a place of suffering is actually a preliminary realization for the path of yoga or, it might be argued, for any serious spiritual practice.[10]

## FROM UNREAL TO REAL

Almost everyone I know who practices yoga says they started practicing because they were in pain of one kind or another. It's logical that spiritual practice would be inspired by unhappiness with our lives. Otherwise, why would we bother? Isn't it the pain that pushes us to seek a deeper understanding or a deeper purpose?

If the pleasures of life were enough to satisfy us, then we would be fulfilled with the temporary joys of money, beauty, and power. And many people are satisfied—until they're not. Eventually, we'll all be stripped bare. Everything will be taken away from us. Either we'll die, or all those we love will die. It's unavoidable. At some point, this loss, and the suffering it brings, may lead to a spiritual awakening. As Bryant mentioned, this is the first Noble Truth of Buddhism, "Life is suffering." This realization can either feel like the burden of a lifetime or weight lifted off our shoulders. The choice is ours.

We can see that living in denial of our mortality is a kind of lie. As Ibram X. Kendi explains, "Lies are like pain relievers, allowing us to momentarily feel better. The painful truth allows us to heal. There's going to be pain regardless. Pain is a part of life. But lies do not have to be."[11] The challenge of yoga is whether we can suffer and be honest with ourselves about why or whether we continue to tell ourselves lies to avoid future suffering.

In fact, in the next sutra, 2.16, Patanjali explains that, "Fortunately, future suffering can be prevented."[12] He goes on to explain that the way we reduce suffering is by cultivating *viveka*, or discriminative discernment, the ability to see clearly between what is permanent or real (purusha) and what is impermanent or unreal (prakriti).

In contemporary Western thinking, we have separated the mind from the body. It was Descartes's fault, when he declared, "I think, therefore I am." This idea, that because we have a mind we exist, is in stark contrast to the way that ancient yogis have envisioned our human embodiment. According to yoga, we are neither the body nor the mind, but instead, pure consciousness. In some systems of yoga, pure consciousness is personified as the god Shiva, who together with the energy of the goddess Shakti, forms the basis of all existence. This duality can also be understood through the terms I mentioned before that Patanjali uses, purusha (spirit) and prakriti (nature).

According to the yoga teachings, prakriti, creation, is made of three kinds of energy known as the *gunas*. These three energies are peaceful energy (*sattva*), excited energy (*rajas*), and lethargic energy (*tamas*). The entire universe is made up of various combinations of these three elements, and so is our body and mind. In fact, the scientists who created quantum theory found much of their inspiration in the ancient yogic teachings.[13] I wonder if the basic concept of protons, neutrons, and electrons can also be connected to the gunas?

Ancient yoga practitioners didn't conceive of our body-mind as separate from nature. In yoga, prakriti includes us. We're not free from the natural world, and all the things we create are part of the natural world as well. Our job as yoga practitioners is to differentiate between what is spirit and what is nature. That's why I sometimes get confused by the way modern yoga practitioners define yoga as the union between body, breath, and mind. According to yoga, those elements have never been separate. The irony in yoga is that we're not so much uniting with spirit, as we are clearly seeing what's not spirit. Yoga, in this sense, isn't really about union—it's about separation. It's cultivating clear vision so that we can see, in stark contrast, what is impermanent—what is not our essential self, from what is.

This idea of clear perception is a major theme in the yoga teachings. It's found in the *Brihadaranyaka Upanishad* from approximately 700 B.C.E.:

*asato ma sad gamaya*
*tamaso ma jyotir gamaya*
*mrityor ma amritam gamaya*

This mantra is often translated to mean: "Lead us from unreal to real, lead us from darkness to the light, lead us from the fear of death to knowledge of immortality." Darkness is the state of ignorance, or identification with the body and mind. But the meaning could also be understood as, "Lead me to the truth of my existence, which is more than this body and mind. I am spirit."

## WISE MIND

This idea of clear perception, viveka, is also important because in the name of meditation—which is perhaps the quintessential yoga practice—we're often taught to force the mind to be quiet. It's as if the mind is something bad that we need to stop or destroy. This leads to a lot of confusion regarding the practice of yoga meditation, and it feeds into self-doubt regarding our ability to practice effectively.

Patanjali actually introduces the eight limbs of yoga (ashtanga yoga) with the clear goal of cultivating viveka. He explains, "By the practice of the limbs of yoga, the impurities dwindle away and there dawns the light of wisdom, leading to discriminative discernment (viveka)."[14] All the teachings we generally think of as yoga—asana, pranayama, and meditation, which are included in the eight limbs—are all taught with the specific goal of cultivating viveka, clear perception.

The point is, yoga is not just about stopping the mind, as Patanjali advocates, at least not unless our goal is renouncing the world. Instead, it's about learning how to use the mind wisely, to cultivate discernment. This may seem like a minor point, but I think it has huge repercussions. We have created modern yoga systems around a philosophy of quietness, calmness, and stillness, which feels misguided for contemporary householder practitioners. Rather, we can engage with our inner wisdom, our wise mind. This is a different kind of empowered practice, where we have the tools within us to find the truth. We don't have to become empty vessels for a teacher or guru to fill us with wisdom.

This idea of wise mind has been used powerfully in the work of Marsha Linehan, PhD, and her school of psychology called Dialectical Behavior Therapy (DBT). It's probably not a coincidence that a dialectic is the ability to hold two seemingly contradictory truths, which is reminiscent of the human condition that Patanjali is describing—being both purusha *and* prakriti.

> Respect your emotion.
> Ask Wise Mind: Which actions will make it better or worse?
> Pain can't be avoided; it is nature's way of signaling that
>     something is wrong.
> Willingness is listening very carefully to your Wise Mind, and
>     then acting from your Wise Mind.
> All people at any given point in time are doing the best they can.
> —MARSHA M. LINEHAN[15]

I sometimes wonder what a yoga practice looks like if it's based on the cultivation of viveka? It would be a practice based in the idea that we already have access to infinite wisdom. Our intuition, that inner knowing, is the element that we can cultivate in our practice. This may be reflected not only in the way we practice meditation, but in the way we practice asana, and all of yoga. Our practice can be built on this foundation of inner knowing, trust, and agency.

Yoga starts with the understanding that we already have what we need inside, we just need to access it. Perhaps we also have the wisdom within us to take us there. What if you consider the idea that all the joy and peace that yoga has given you has come from you, that you are the source? Think of every Shavasana, every conscious exhale, each moment of peace, every pause in your endless ruminating, every asana that has created space in your joints and the release of muscle bound tension. What if you took full responsibility for those experiences and realized that they are truly yours, and a reflection of what lies within you? No one gave them to you.

The next time you step on your mat, see what it feels like to start with the thought, "I know," instead of the idea, "I don't know." Or the next time you sit in meditation, start with the thought, "I have truth within me, and my work is to remove the obstacles to that inner wisdom, and uncover that truth." An intuitive yoga practice looks very different than the practice most of us are experiencing these days in contemporary yoga.

Intuitive practice values the messages that are constantly arising from the body and mind. We don't need to push them away with meditation techniques that work like dog training: "Bad mind!" Instead, ask your mind, "What is bothering you? Let's find the way through. How can we build this life together? Let me listen to you and work with you to sharpen our vision to serve ourself and others."

This is an idea we'll explore further in the last section of the book as we look at how to build an effective yoga practice. But it's important to sit with this question in all aspects of our lives, on and off the mat: How can I cultivate intuition and trust my inner wisdom?

> Rather than focusing on stillness, take a moment to sit with yourself and try to connect to the energy of your mind. Encourage your mind to be active, and ask yourself, "How can I cultivate clear vision?" "How can I connect to my inner knowing?" "How can I work with my mind instead of against it?"

# 3 | CONNECTING TO THE SOURCE OF THE TEACHINGS

THE GAYATRI MANTRA, A PRAYER FOR ENLIGHTENMENT
*om bhur bhuva svah*
*tat savitur varenyam*
*bhargo devasya dhimahi*
*dhiyo yo nah prachodayat*

Heaven, earth, and all between.
May we contemplate the radiant power
Of the sun's divine light and energy;
May this inspire our understanding.[1]

—RIG VEDA 3.62.10

THE GAYATRI MANTRA reaches us across the expanse of time and space. This sacred mantra is found in the Rig Veda, one of the oldest known Sanskrit texts, which may be over 3,500 years old. The message of the Gayatri is a celebration of light, enlightenment, and clarity. According to the professor of religion Douglas Brooks, "the Gayatri is the most sacred phrase uttered in the Vedas."[2] The Gayatri is also mentioned in the Bhagavad Gita:

I am the beginning, middle, and end of creation.
I am infinite time, and the sustainer whose face is seen
    everywhere. I am death, which overcomes all, and the
    source of all beings still to be born.
Among poetic meters, the Gayatri.
Among seasons I am spring, that brings forth flowers.
I am the silence of the unknown and the wisdom of the wise.

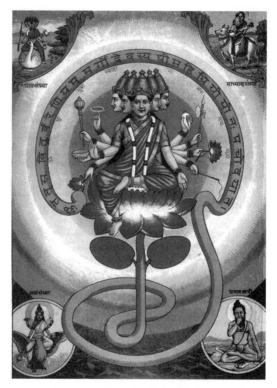

A representation of the Gayatri mantra as
a goddess by Raja Ravi Varna (1848–1906)[3]

> I am the seed that can be found in every creature, Arjuna;
> for without me nothing can exist, neither animate nor
> inanimate.[4]

Swami Vivekananda distilled the message of the Gayatri in this way:
"We meditate on the glory of that Being who has produced this universe;
may She enlighten our minds."[5] This is a prayer for clear vision and clear
understanding, which can arise through mantra repetition. Yet most contemporary yoga practitioners spend little time directly studying scripture or
reciting traditional mantra. Rather, we rely on our yoga teachers to decipher
them for us or to share their personal experiences. Part of our practice can
be a journey back to the source of the teachings to reflect on their meaning
in our lives right now.

Repeating a mantra for an extended period of time allows different levels of its meaning to appear. There is the power of the sound vibration, the way it feels in the body, and the effect it has on the breath and the mind. There is also the meaning of the words and how we relate to that meaning: in this case, a sense of gratitude to the immensity and brilliance of all creation.

With the Gayatri mantra there is a feeling greater than just gratitude. It's a feeling of pure respect and a sense of surrender to the wisdom of the universe that is so much greater than our individual ego-mind. The humility that comes from this kind of an open, pure relationship with creation establishes our ability to listen to the messages from the spiritual realm. Remember, these are messages that arise from the depth of our own being. The spiritual realm isn't somewhere out there. It's closer than our own heart.

Try to repeat the Gayatri mantra, with a focus on its meaning. Consider what it feels like to have your mind filled with the light of wisdom. If you're not familiar with the Gayatri, try looking up audio versions of the mantra to hear correct pronunciation.

## REFLECTIONS ON MY TEACHERS

My connection to the teachings has been greatly affected by my relationship with my teacher, Swami Satchidananda. Recently, I've been reflecting on the way that relationship has shifted and changed over the years. It's a long and complicated relationship, and like any student, it's matured as I've grown.

Some of my earliest childhood memories are of my grandmother practicing yoga each morning. She would do a series of asanas every day, which was even more remarkable because she must have already been in her sixties by that time. I remember her patiently teaching me alternate-nostril breathing to a one-two count: inhale one and exhale two. Mostly, I just loved spending time with her, and that made yoga seem so much more compelling. She would often practice with a book next to her that had a mesmerizing cover. It was the face of Swami Satchidananda in gold on his book *Integral Yoga Hatha*.

That image of his gold face must have stayed with me, because decades later, in 1990, it appeared again. I was getting a massage to help me deal with the burnout I was experiencing from my activism, and the massage therapist, Kazuko Onodera, had a picture of Swami Satchidananda on her wall. I remember saying to her, "I think I know that guy." And she said, "Yes, he's my yoga teacher. You should come to my yoga classes and meet him when he comes to town." So I did. I began taking classes with her religiously, and she started training me to be a yoga teacher.

Little did I realize, I had stumbled upon a rich yoga tradition and a powerful teacher in Kazuko. She took me on as an apprentice, and I spent many years studying by her side. She taught me how to garden, how to cook, how to practice yoga, and how to integrate the teachings into my life. It was the best training I could have wished for, at the exact moment when I desperately needed a mentor.

In 1991, Kazuko eventually brought me to meet Swami Satchidananda in person when he gave a public talk in San Francisco. When I first met him, I was impressed with his tremendous knowledge of yoga and yogic scriptures. I enjoyed his humor, especially his endless puns. But I was confused by the reactions of the people around him, by their devotion, and the religious feeling of the gathering.

I was a young, queer, AIDS activist fighting against a system of oppression that was killing my friends. I couldn't easily accept another authority figure because I felt that this kind of hierarchical thinking was at the basis of our problems. I even found some homophobic quotes from Swami Satchidananda, which totally turned me off.

But I soon found myself surrounded by an amazing community of yoga practitioners who touched me with the passion they felt for yoga, and I was mesmerized by the teachings themselves, which answered so many of my big life questions. I soon learned that Swami Satchidananda had changed his mind about the homophobic remarks, and I was even invited to help edit one of his books to take out those sections and make the language more inclusive.

I slowly got involved at the San Francisco Integral Yoga Institute, and there I found a family of yoga practitioners—a sangha, or spiritual community—to support me in my practice. I was desperate for answers and felt so drawn to the teachings. But it was the support of this community that propelled me forward through study, intensive practice, shared conversations, and general camaraderie.

## APPRECIATION AND DISAPPOINTMENT

In 1997, my partner, Matt, and I started talking about having a commitment ceremony. I was excited by the idea of having this ceremony at my spiritual home, the Integral Yoga Institute. This was years before anyone was talking about gay marriage, so it was still very unusual. I was told to ask Swami Satchidananda in person when he next visited. When the time came, I was very nervous. I had spoken to him on only a few occasions, and he was this very intense, wise yogi.

I stood in line to speak to him, and when it was my turn, I asked him if Matt and I could get married at the Institute. He responded by asking me, "When?" I said, "August 31," embarrassed that we had already scheduled a date before we got his approval. He simply said, "Of course." Then about half an hour later after talking to a long line of people, he approached me and said, "I'll be thinking of you on August 31." He even wrote us a note that was read at the ceremony, which said, "Have a blessed matrimonial life."

His acceptance of our gay marriage was exactly what I needed to assuage any of my concerns about getting more involved and making a personal commitment to him and his teachings. In 2001, I deepened my commitment to yoga, and to serving in the name of the yoga teachings, by being ordained as an Integral Yoga Minister. The ministry was created by Swami Satchidananda as a way for householders to take a vow that was similar to the monastic vows that are traditional in yoga lineages.

When I first asked about becoming a minister, I was met with concern from a few senior members of the organization who worried that having a gay minister was inappropriate. Once again, I had to approach Swami Satchidananda directly. I remember speaking with him as he was walking onstage to give a talk. I told him I was interested in becoming a minister, and he stopped and asked me, "Are you sure?" I responded, "Yes." Then he whacked me hard on the back, between my shoulder blades, and said, "Okay."

I now see how that commitment was a mixed blessing. On a personal level, it allowed me to go deeper with my practice. I felt guided by him and clear in my mission of nonattachment and service. But, as I got more involved, I would always ask a lot of questions and often the answers were vague.

I heard that there was a group of women protesting at one of his talks in New York City in the early 1990s. They accused him of a pattern of sexual misconduct and of silencing their voices. When I inquired more about it, I was told that these women were basically projecting their own problems onto him. The sad part is that I believed that story at the time.

The #MeToo movement helped me understand the way that sexual abuse works and how these women's voices were silenced. I now have a different perspective on the situation, and I'm devastated that I wasn't able to help make their voices heard. As I have more time to reflect on my relationship with Swami Satchidananda, I see his brilliance and also his flaws.

The question, as usual, is whether we can apply the yoga teachings in the turbulent moments of our lives or if we retreat to a defensive position focused on protecting our need to be right. This is the tension that is at the heart of our practice: am I loving and compassionate, or am I dedicated to protecting my personal belief system (the samskaras and attachments in my mind)? This represents the transformational potential of yoga and a more accessible and practically helpful understanding of samadhi, freedom from the prison of our own thoughts.

It's important to understand that fundamental truths are not the same as beliefs. The truth is that Black lives matter, that everyone deserves basic human rights no matter their ability or background. Human rights are a universal truth, not a belief. So the movement for social justice is not a question of standing up for what I believe, it's a matter of protecting certain unalienable human rights. So, the question here, regarding Swami Satchidananda, isn't really about what did or didn't happen, but how I can affirm the rights of those who feel like they are powerless.

For a long time, I struggled with how to reconcile my gratitude for what I learned from Swami Satchidananda, and for the kind and generous way he treated me personally, with what I heard about the way he treated these women. My job is to practice ahimsa, actively loving everyone and standing up for their rights—especially if they were disempowered or abused. It's also my job to participate in creating a yoga community where abuse no longer happens, and when it does it gets called out and addressed immediately.

Mostly, I realized that I couldn't keep parts of my life separate—ethics need to be universally applied. That is one way that we clearly see the way that yoga is political. Yoga ethics require that we integrate all aspects of our lives. These

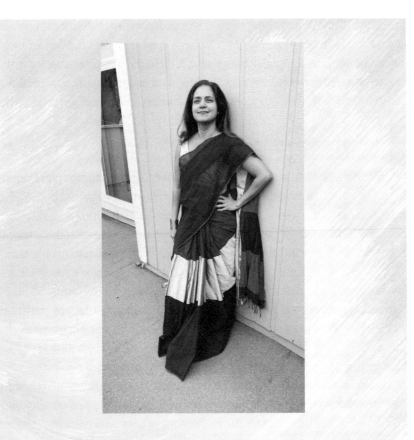

### ANJALI RAO

Yoga and social justice work deeply intersect one another. One may ask, "But how is this connected to yoga? Isn't yoga about peace and oneness? How is the revolution for social and racial justice an extension of our practice?" I believe that the work of social justice is itself the very essence of our practice; our yoga practice is deeply embedded in the world around us. It is a mirror, a microcosm, of the world outside. Our inner lives are connected to the way we move in the world, our relationships with one another, how we practice integrity, speak truth in our work and community around us. We learn this as students of the Yoga Sutras, the yamas and the niyamas. We learn this from the ancient Upanishads. We learn this from the Bhagavad Gita.

are not concepts that can be applied haphazardly or when they are convenient. Even though I owe so much to my teacher, I can't disregard the concerns expressed about him. As Anjali Rao explains, "Our inner lives are connected to the way we move in the world, our relationships with one another, how we practice integrity, speak truth in our work and community around us."

## THE GURU-DISCIPLE RELATIONSHIP NOW

I know firsthand that there is tremendous power in the guru-disciple relationship, but I think we've overstated its importance in the yoga tradition. We've muddied the role of a good teacher with the power of devotion—bhakti yoga. Swami Satchidananda was the person who shared these incredible teachings with me, and I will always be incredibly grateful for what he taught me. But, I also consider my grandmother, Kazuko, AIDS activists, my students, my husband and children, and many other people to be my gurus. So many people have supported me along the way, and I owe them a debt of gratitude.

Bhakti yoga—the yoga of devotion, which includes devotion to the guru—is such a powerful group of yoga practices because it allows practitioners to engage their emotions. It also offers the benefit of dedicating your actions to someone or something else, releasing us from the grip of the ego. But the risks of this type of devotion to any single, fallible person outweigh the benefits. In the yoga tradition, the guru is seen as a manifestation of God. So, many people defend their teacher at whatever cost because they are defending the essence of the guru.

I don't think we need to discard these practices altogether. Rather they can evolve and grow as the yoga community evolves. Instead of focusing our bhakti love toward the guru, we can focus that energy toward the teachings themselves, or the community. In fact, I specifically remember Swami Satchidananda telling us not to look to him, but to the teachings, as the guru. We can hold on to the guru principle—*guru tattva*, the essence of the teacher—the lineage, and the teachings.

> Ask yourself if there is a special teacher or figure in your life that you feel especially grateful for. What was the special quality that person found in you? Can you identify that quality in yourself and take responsibility for it?

Bhakti practices include chanting, praying, prostrating, having an altar and finding images that represent the divine. It's also important to note that the relationship between bhakti yoga and karma yoga, selfless action, is profound. It's really impossible to be of service if love isn't your motivating factor. Whatever service we offer in the world needs to be based on love, either love for the people you are serving or for the activity itself.

As we move into a time of post-lineage yoga, I think we should celebrate our independence from traditional gurus who were so often abusive. But we can keep in mind that there were benefits to the guru relationship that may be lost—the power of tradition and lineage, the focused attention, the individual support—but this should not keep us from seeing how the mentorship of the guru can be cultivated in new ways. Within yoga communities, we can replace the power of the guru with the support of the collective and explore the benefits of devotion, service, and dedication to each other.

As yoga teachers, we have a shared responsibility to lift each other up, to educate each other, and to help each other do better. But it needs to come from a place of care, not a place of competition. If we can let go of the weight of capitalism—always doing more and being more—we can open ourselves to others in our community whom we can support, and who will support us in exchange. Perhaps this takes the form of a mentorship program, or maybe it's a teachers' group, a book group, or a teachers' workshop. Maybe it means reaching out to teachers you know and asking them how you can support them or how you can support each other. It seems to me that this kind of peer mentoring is one of the missing pieces in contemporary yoga practice.

We can also look to nature as our guru. In so many ways, the trees have more wisdom than we do, not to mention the ocean and all its inhabitants, the wind and the way it sings. There is tremendous wisdom all around us, if we just look.

# 4 | EMBODYING THE EIGHT LIMBS OF YOGA

RECENTLY, A GROUP OF scientists proposed that the octopus may actually be an alien species.[1] They are suggesting that the genetic makeup of the octopus family is so foreign from any other animal on earth that there is a good chance they have alien ancestry. Possibly, some of their genes came to earth on a meteor—in essence bringing life from another planet. So many horror movies and sci-fi adventures explore the idea of alien invaders. It's hard to imagine that the men from Mars that we fear could simply be the octopus swimming around in our oceans.

How is it possible that something as ordinary as an octopus can be so alien? You could say the same thing about yoga. It's such an ordinary part of life: What's more common these days than seeing a person wearing yoga pants carrying a yoga mat walking down the street? But the essential philosophy of yoga is completely foreign to Western culture and the systems that we hold so dear. Unfortunately, yoga has been appropriated by Western culture, and the essence of the teachings can hardly be found in our contemporary practice.

The heart of yoga denies all the tenets of capitalism. So instead of embracing a philosophy that's so foreign and different, we tend to pick apart yoga like a dead octopus, and the practice we offer in the West ends up more like calamari, just small fried pieces of what was once a complex and gorgeous living being. We pretend that complicated yoga poses are the goal of an ancient spiritual tradition that focused on subduing the ego rather than emboldening it.

I'm not criticizing people who love yoga just for the poses. I love the poses too. But how do we excuse our fear of the deeper spiritual teachings? How do we avoid answering the challenging questions of yoga? Why are we satisfied wading in the shallows with Fish Pose and Dolphin Pose? (Yes, this is stretching an analogy, but the origin story of yoga takes place at the bottom of the ocean, where Lord Matsyendra was living inside the belly of a fish and overheard the secrets of yoga being shared by Shiva.)

## A FOSSILIZED WORLDVIEW

The famous bhakti poet Hafiz said it succinctly: "The world has its pants on backwards." To truly embrace yoga, we need to accept that our fundamental understanding and perception of the world may be screwed up. And who is willing to do that? I know that for me it's scary, and something I tend to avoid. When I was younger it was different. I spent lots of time in meditation, on retreats, reading scripture, and actually challenging the perceptions of my mind and the way I experience the world around me.

But, as I get older and my responsibilities grow, like raising children, making mortgage payments, and so on, I notice my worldview has fossilized. I've created a pattern of beliefs that allow me to get through the day. I don't usually have time to challenge my fundamental understanding of things, I'm too busy answering email and planning for my next class.

To live in the question is a very difficult thing to do, but that's what yoga demands. Yoga isn't afraid to ask us who we really are. Are we the mind and the constantly changing thoughts, or are we the consciousness that's simply observing? Are we in the game playing, or are we standing on the sidelines like a referee?

Sometimes in meditation, I can see a thought for what it is. I hear the words simply as words, rather than focusing on their meaning. In order to see my thoughts as thoughts, I have to identify with another part of myself. I have to connect to that witness: the observer. Not taking sides, not allowing the mind to obsess over wins and losses. As Swami Sivananda used to say, "Likes and dislikes, that's the problem." Or as explained in the Bhagavad Gita:

> When your mind, which has been tossed about by conflicting opinions, becomes still and centered in equilibrium, then you experience Yoga.[2]

Maybe I'm just jaded, or having a yoga midlife crisis, but I have noticed this same tendency in those around me. We no longer expect transcendental moments in our practice. Instead, we search for a hint of sanity in a world that often feels out of control. Have we lowered our expectations too much?

In the Yoga Sutras, Patanjali explains that future suffering is avoidable, as I described earlier, and to avoid suffering we need to cultivate discriminative discernment (viveka) to distinguish what is permanent (purusha) and what is impermanent (prakriti). Patanjali goes on to say that discriminative discernment, viveka, is cultivated by practicing the eight limbs (let's call them tentacles) of yoga.

The eight limbs of yoga are:
1. Yama
2. Niyama
3. Asana
4. Pranayama
5. Pratyahara
6. Dharana
7. Dhyana
8. Samadhi[3]

## PERSONALIZING SYSTEMIC PROBLEMS

To give some context to the eight limbs, it's important to note that Patanjali has just described the obstacles to our enlightenment (the *kleshas*) as well as explained how karma works. It can be depressing and overwhelming to honestly face the challenges of the human condition. Enlightenment may feel like an unattainable goal, but reducing our suffering seems reachable and even essential for our survival.

Of course, one of the dangers of yoga is that we are personalizing a systemic problem. How much of our suffering is caused by societal discrimination and oppression of all kinds? Are we responsible for the racism, sexism, or homophobia that we endure? Sure, future suffering is avoidable, but changing the systems that add to that suffering is also essential.

In many ways, Patanjali offers us a path for changing these harmful systems. They're found in the very first limb of ashtanga yoga: yama (abstinence). Yama is a group of five ethical teachings, things not to do: *ahimsa*, not causing suffering; *satya*, not lying; *asteya*, not stealing, *brahmacharya*, not wasting resources; and *aparigraha*, not being greedy.

If we practiced these five ethical values as a society we would be rid of most forms of oppression. These teachings can be understood another way. In the United States, yama could be practiced the following way to undo centuries of harm and create an environment that is ripe for racial and social reconciliation.

1. Ahimsa—Caring for everyone equally; universal health care and human rights
2. Satya—Honest reconciliation with the sins of the past, including racism
3. Asteya—Reparations for slavery and for land and resources stolen from Native communities
4. Brahmacharya—Preserving natural resources and caring for the earth
5. Aparigraha—Sharing resources and power with Black, Indigenous, and People of Color (BIPOC) as well as other marginalized groups.

## A WAY OUT OF SUFFERING

Next, Patanjali offers the five niyamas, or "observances," which can be viewed as active practices to find our way out of suffering. Niyama includes *shaucha*, purity; *santosha*, contentment; *tapas*, learning from suffering; *svadhyaya,* reflection; and *ishvarapranidhana*, surrender to God. It's worth noting that *ishvara* isn't exactly God, as we conceive of it. Ishvara is more about your highest self, or what the scholar Shyam Ranganathan describes as becoming your ideal person.[4]

Niyama are all big ideas, and in some way each of them can be seen as a microcosm for the entirety of yoga teachings. For example, santosha, being content with what is, seems like a form of enlightenment, a state of total acceptance and peace. It's also important to note that the last three, tapas, svadhyaya, and ishvarapranidhana, which I discussed earlier, are repeated here after Patanjali offers them in the very first sutra of chapter 2, the portion on practice.

After offering these teachings, Patanjali inserts an interesting tool: *pratipaksha bhavana*, "positive thinking." Actually that's a simplified definition. Patanjali explains that pratipaksha bhavana can mean replacing negative thoughts, or it can be a process of reflecting on negative thinking and understanding that it eventually leads to suffering.

> Upon being harassed by negative thoughts, one should cultivate counteracting thoughts. Negative thoughts are violence, etc. They may be [personally] performed, performed on one's behalf by another, or authorized by oneself; they may be triggered by greed, anger, or delusion; and they may be slight, moderate, or extreme in intensity. One should cultivate counteracting thoughts, namely, that the end results [of negative thoughts] are ongoing suffering and ignorance.[5]

This is an important idea, since he's just explained that yoga offers an end to suffering and a way to avoid future pain. For example, if you're lying in bed at night angry about something someone said to you, the question eventually arises: are you making the situation worse, or is that obsessive thinking actually addressing the problem? Probably, it's just reducing the quality of your sleep and negatively affecting your health. In other words, it's bringing ongoing suffering.

Patanjali offers pratipaksha bhavana after yama and niyama to show that the teachings of niyama are the positive action needed to address the challenges he just exposed. In a way, tapas sets the stage for the entire section on practicing yoga. As I see it, tapas is the acknowledgment that we are suffering, and svadhyaya asks us why. Eventually, you find that the answer is always the same. It's because you haven't trusted yourself, which is what ishvarapranidhana really means. Trust your own heart, and know that is where your peace truly lives.

As I mentioned before, your suffering may be the result of external forces over which you have no control. But what can you control? How can you take care of yourself in a way that fills you up and makes you stronger for the challenges of the world? That's what Patanjali is offering us: self-care in the form of ethical values, practical tools, and effective practices to reduce our suffering.

Headstands are fun, but are they reducing your pain or increasing it? That's the question of the third limb of yoga, asana, or posture. Interestingly, Patanjali explains that asana is a steady, comfortable pose, and that the way to practice asana is to work against the mind's natural tendency for restlessness

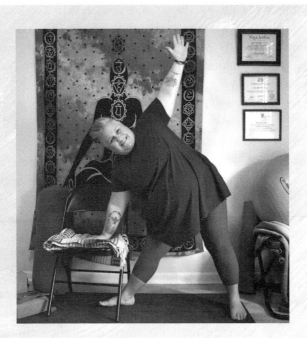

### JACQUIE SUNNY BARBEE

Through my practice of svadhyaya—self-study—I'm able to connect my yoga practice and social justice work to propel inner and social change. Justice and equity work are deep, and it's impossible to make lasting changes without becoming aware of my own internalized biases and privileges as a white person. I lean into the ugly truths and injustices, working for change rather than spiritually bypassing.

I also try to create space in my yoga classes for students to be their most authentic self, where they can safely move through their own personal life challenges and traumas with their practice. As a plus-sized practitioner living with chronic illness I am able to show that yoga truly is for everyone and that all asana can be made accessible by exploring different variations of each pose. My classes are a place where people of all sizes, ages, abilities, race, and gender identity can feel safe and form a deeper, more loving relationship with their bodies. Together we celebrate what our bodies can do.

by meditating on the infinite. I'm not sure how often that concept is taught in most yoga classes, but it's a powerful and intriguing directive.

As we move our body into shapes (or sit in meditation) we can settle the mind by focusing on something: the breath, a point inside the body, a point outside the body, energy, or sensations. Focusing the mind and working on stability and stillness are how asana is practiced (nothing about extreme flexibility or strength is mentioned).

Of course, in this context, Patanjali was thinking of asana as "seat," a cross-legged position for meditation. After finding a comfortable seat, Patanjali offers the fourth limb, pranayama. *Prana* means energy or life force, and *ayama* is control. So a definition of *pranayama* would include working with the breath to control or calm internal energy. He goes on to say that the practice of *pranayama* can remove the veil over the inner light, which feels like a form of realization in itself.

The fifth limb of ashtanga yoga is *pratyahara*, sense withdrawal, or moving away from external influences. I like to think of pratyahara as vritti prevention. Previously, Patanjali told us that yoga is about restraining the vrittis, or thoughts, in the mind. But where do all these thoughts come from? They all come through the senses, so it makes sense that turning our awareness within would help calm the mind and prepare for meditation.

Pratyahara is also the beginning of formal seated meditation, and it's the step that is most often overlooked on the journey of the eight limbs. When we go sit in meditation we are already withdrawing the senses. We sit in one place, turn off our phone, close the door, and ask our family not to disturb us. These are all efforts to restrict sensory input. Pratyahara is a very practical yoga tool. It is a matter of increased awareness of the impact of sensory stimuli on our nervous system and our mind.

The other night my husband and I were watching a movie that was very intense and disturbing. At one point, I realized that my heart was racing, and the film was upsetting me. I didn't quite have the energy to go on that roller-coaster ride, so I went into the other room. I realized that I was allowing my mind to be stimulated by my senses in experiencing that movie. It wasn't a bad thing, but it was something I did have control of in that moment. So, instead, I chose to find an activity that was less disturbing. There are enough real-life events that disturb me. I don't need extra ones from movies (unless it's science fiction)!

The next time you are watching or reading something that disturbs you, see if you can take a pause and notice its impact on your nervous system and on your mind.

## FROM CONCENTRATION TO MEDITATION

In the beginning of chapter 3, Patanjali offers the sixth limb, *dharana*, or concentration. Concentration is the key to meditation in the yoga system. This is a slightly different focus than mindfulness, which has become synonymous with meditation in contemporary spiritual practices. With mindfulness we try to step outside our thoughts into the role of the witness. Although the goal of both practices may be the same, dharana offers a slightly different direction by concentrating the mind on a neutral object, such as a mantra. Or, as Patanjali offers in sutra 1.39, one can concentrate on any place, object, or idea (basically anything!).

Actually, I think that's an important point to emphasize. Patanjali is saying we can focus on any object that we choose. What he is offering us is a technique free from the restraints of a specific religious dogma. In a few places, he does recommend repeating the sacred sound of OM as a way to focus the mind and destroy the obstacles to our enlightenment. But here, he defines the practice as the act of concentration itself, regardless of the object upon which you have chosen to concentrate.

I also wonder if concentration is always about making the mind smaller and laser focused. In my experience, there is a process of widening the focus, accepting all, that is most effective and differs from limiting my mind. Instead, I challenge my mind to include everything without preference or prejudice—to welcome everything. It reminds me of the way that something moving incredibly fast looks like it's standing still.

Experiment with practicing a meditation that invites the mind to welcome all thoughts, ideas, emotions, and images. Take a moment to turn within and observe how active your mind is. Try saying the word "yes" every time some new thought appears. Notice if welcoming the thoughts, rather than pushing them away, can create a sense of calm and peace.

The seventh limb, *dhyana*, is meditation, or the flow state. Dhyana is usually understood as a deepening of concentration, where the mind becomes completely focused on the object of meditation in an unbroken stream of thought. This flow state is described by athletes, artists, musicians, and performers of all kinds. It's a state of mind that allows us to transcend the limitations of space and time. We become absorbed in the present moment in a way that lifts us out of the self-consciousness of ego. Again, it's a process of expanding beyond normal limitations.

It's important to note that meditation is a natural state that is fundamental to our creative spirit. You could think of it as the way to work with your own mind to cultivate creativity. In fact, you could say that creativity is spirituality. Why do we pursue certain hobbies or the arts? Making music, painting, writing, dancing, or creating anything connects us to the energy of creation. It's also interesting to consider how meditation and creativity connect to self-discipline.

Without structure it's hard to be creative. If I'm an untrained pianist, my improvisation will be horrible. But once I have some mastery on the instrument, through disciplined practice, I can improvise and be more creative. The thing is that creative pursuits don't always work to focus the mind, and we may find ourselves in a dry spell. But yoga is designed to cultivate this flow state. In fact, everything that we do in the name of yoga eventually leads us to meditation in one form or another.

Essentially, all the practices of yoga are about calming the mind through focus and attention. Sometimes this is done consciously, through classical meditation, and sometimes it's a side benefit, maybe through asana or chanting. In the end, yoga practices create the environment where the state of meditation, dhyana, can happen spontaneously. I've offered a few other approaches to meditation in the practice prompts scattered through this book, as well as in the last chapter on building your own practice. I hope you'll explore them to see if there is a technique that is effective for you.

Sustained meditation is samadhi, enlightenment, the eighth limb of ashtanga yoga. Samadhi may seem out of reach, the state of Buddha or other enlightened masters. But what if it's not? What if samadhi is a place that spontaneously arises in moments of joy and bliss? My sense is that samadhi is the most natural of all our experiences, the core of our being, our heart of hearts. In many ways, this is what Patanjali has been urging us to do from the very beginning—connect with our own true self. Samadhi is the end of separation and ego. It can lead to the end of identification with the body and mind, and an expansion of consciousness to include all other beings; it is universal compassion, deep service, and expansive love.

In ashtanga yoga, Patanjali offers a step-by-step method for cultivating discrimination and clear perception. The steps are directed inward to detach us from the world, but the clear vision we gain can help us see through the mist of ego and the ways we have created separation and harm. The limbs don't have to be practiced in order, but they are all effective tools for our journey toward self-awareness. Simply put, yoga is about seeing ourselves clearly, cleaning up the messes we have made, and then reducing harm in the world.

# 5 | RAINBOW MIND: ENLIGHTENMENT TODAY

THE FIRST RULE OF yoga is ahimsa, which means nonviolence or non-harm. But what is nonviolence? Is it the opposite of violence? If so, wouldn't you say the opposite of violence is love—an active engaged love? I suggest that social justice is actually a manifestation of ahimsa in which we practice an engaged love. Ahimsa is expressing our love for each other, for animals, and for the earth by speaking out against injustice, violence, and harm. According to a translation of the Yoga Sutras by one of my teachers, Nischala Joy Devi, ahimsa can be understood as reverence and love. She translates sutra 2:35 as, "Embracing reverence and love for all (*ahimsa*), we experience oneness."[1]

Matthew Remski takes up this point in his creative translation of the Yoga Sutras:

> If we're going to continue using this text in contemporary yoga culture, we must acknowledge the vacuum of love—in whatever way we use the term today—at its centre, and recognize that we have voices where Patanjali is silent. Perhaps we can start by reversing the purpose of his ethical discussion, so that our intention behind treating others kindly is not about internal equanimity, but about the exploration of empathy as a path to self-and-other growth.[2]

As Amber Karnes explains (see sidebar), our practice is an opportunity to remember that we're not as separate from other people as we like to imagine. Engaging in social justice movements is a way of putting that understanding into practice by offering love and compassion to those who have been harmed, including ourselves. Marching for people with AIDS, or for Black lives, is an expression of love and care. In fact, it is our duty,

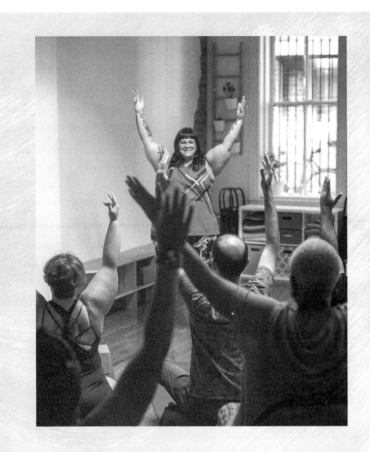

**AMBER KARNES**

Dominant culture conditions us to forget our own humanity and function as "every man for himself." My yoga practice helps me to remember that I am not separate from my humanity or from other people in this world. The yoga teachings speak to our interconnectedness and remind me that my actions have a ripple effect on others. And so my yoga practice is a journey of liberation (of my own heart, mind, body, and spirit). This yogic journey of turning attention inward isn't about becoming self-obsessed, but rather remembering my own humanity so that I may see the same in others and then be of service toward liberation and justice.

our dharma, to protect and love those who are suffering. The writer and activist adrienne maree brown describes the way her activism intersects with spirituality in her seminal book, *Emergent Strategy*:

> In all these ways, I meditate on love. This practice lets me connect to the part of myself that is divine, aligned with the universe, and the place within myself where I can be a conduit for spiritual truth—I don't know what else to call it. What comes forth, as lessons and realizations and beliefs—doesn't feel political, or even about organizing. It feels like spirit leading me to the truth.[3]

Is our activism the outgrowth of love or hate? Sometimes it's hard to tell the difference because our love for our community can make us angry when its members are suffering. In many ways, that's what happened to me during the AIDS crisis. I acted out of love, but I also became bitterly angry that the world would disregard the suffering of my friends and community. Anger helped motivate me to become an activist, to march in the street, and to stand my ground. I couldn't have done all of those intense and scary things without anger, so I honor it.

## THE GOAL OF YOGA

If the first rule of yoga, ahimsa, is engaged love, then what is the goal of yoga? Often the goal of yoga is described by one word: s*amadhi*. The word is often translated as "enlightenment," a kind of transcendent meditative state that, to be honest, most of us don't even aspire to, at least not in the way it's currently understood.

Patanjali explains that, "When the object of meditation only shines forth in the mind, as though devoid of the thought of even the self (who is meditating), that state is called samadhi or concentration." The original commentary on the sutras, expands further on this teaching: "When the state of meditation (dhyana) becomes so deep that only the object stands by itself, obliterating, as it were, all traces of reflective thought, it is known as samadhi."[4] This basically means that the ego-mind has disappeared. The object is shining because it can be experienced in its truth, its essence is revealed. The mind is no longer interpreting or translating it.

It's similar to the experience of listening to someone speak through a translator, versus listening to them speak in a language you are fluent in. You have to wonder how much of the translator's mind is being shared. Is it possible to completely understand what the original speaker is saying? Can we experience reality without the ego-mind filtering it? What would it be like to experience life objectively rather than subjectively?

Patanjali explains that we are experiencing the natural world through the colored lens of our attachments. We are constantly interpreting and deciphering the messages we get through our senses. But samadhi is a neutral state, where our mind's influence disappears; it is perfectly clear vision. This is what I like to call, "rainbow mind," pure clarity and neutrality, accepting all and loving all without prejudice. This is a mind that is so expansive it's as wide as a rainbow, and also willing to accept and celebrate difference.

> Find a comfortable position, and take a moment to notice your surroundings. Close your eyes if that's comfortable for you (or leave them open to read this).
>
> Begin to notice all the stimuli you're receiving through your senses. Notice light and color through the eyes, sound through the ears, sensations on the skin, smells, and tastes. Then turn the awareness within and notice inner sensations: pain or discomfort, relaxation or ease, breath, emotions, and thoughts.
>
> Picture a rainbow with a spectrum of color and imagine all these sensations as colors along that spectrum. See if you can allow your mind to embrace all the experiences you're having at this moment, both good and bad. Embrace the sensations, the thoughts, the emotions. Accept every part of yourself as part of this rainbow spectrum.
>
> Take a moment to appreciate how spectacular your rainbow is, with each hue adding to its beauty. Notice how the nuances and differences are what make it so beautiful. Pause and ask yourself: "Can I completely accept myself as I am just for this moment?"

## OPENING THE MIND

With this perspective, we can approach samadhi in a way that speaks to our contemporary lives. In my thinking, samadhi is liberation—true freedom. It's freedom from the limitations of our self-centeredness. We let go of the need for fulfillment from anyone or anything; instead, we become firmly grounded in that space in our own heart that is the center of our consciousness.

After all, the heart is guiding us, not the head. It produces an electromagnetic signal thousands of times stronger than the brain.[5] In fact, one of the benefits of inverted poses extolled by yoga teachers is allowing the heart to be above the head—allowing the heart to lead. There is even a new branch of Western medicine called "neurocardiology," which explores this relationship between the head and the heart.[6]

Traditionally, samadhi is described in very technical terms. In fact, in the first chapter of the Yoga Sutras, Patanjali describes the esoteric levels of samadhi in detail. In later texts on physical practice, samadhi is understood to be the result of the movement of energy, or prana, along the spine. The prana moves through the chakras, expanding each center of wisdom that exists within us, until our mind reflects that level of awareness. This energy work is usually the result of decades of practicing asana, pranayama, and meditation and results from personal discipline and sacrifice.

But I don't think enlightenment is a state completely out of reach for us; rather, it's a state we can find by reaching within us. It's the state we find when we are filled with compassion and love for others, rather than simply focusing on what we want or what we get. This kind of enlightenment feels like the culmination of a life filled with yoga: a life filled with contemplation, meditation, asana, service, and nonattachment. Or is it just the beginning? According to the yoga teacher and Buddhist Michael Stone:

> A single experience of samadhi does not mark the end of practice; it is only the beginning of waking up to the world around us, where spontaneous benevolence of the heart replaces self-centered action. With the understanding of the profound kinship we have with all of life, our spiritual life, our psychological and physical existence, and the choices we make create a seamless mode of being in and of the world. Ethics, psychology, and spirituality are seen to be ongoing, evolving, and interdependent, ensuring that our practice does not go stale.[7]

## MY LIBERATION IS TIED TO YOURS

This practice of liberation is ongoing, and extremely challenging. We get to practice stepping back from the tyranny of our own ego-centered thinking. We also get to step back from a culture we've been steeped in, from a world focused on the individual self, into a life focused on the communality. Liberation is a state of isolation from personal likes and dislikes so that we can get over ourselves. It reminds me of that famous saying by J. Krishnamurti, "Do you want to know my secret? I don't mind what happens." Think of how much freedom that brings.

This can be a hard message to swallow in a culture that teaches us to pursue the fulfillment of all our various desires. Isn't that the main message of our capitalist system? Pursue your dreams at any expense. The question of yoga is, "How can I transcend my personal desires to connect to a universal experience of connection and the communal liberation of all beings?"

This is how my liberation is tied to yours. It's not simply because I'm a nice person, or I'm politically correct. Our hearts are all knotted together in the expanse of space and time. My ability to let go of my personal desires draws me closer and closer to you. As I release myself, I can embrace you more fully. It reminds me of recent scientific research into the substantial similarities between neuronal networks in our brains and the cosmic network of galaxies in the universe—between microcosm and macrocosm.[8] What I find within myself is found without me too.

For example, if we're friends and we have an argument, how do I heal that pain? Say we have both expressed our positions clearly, but we're still stuck in the anger and frustration. Do I stay in my desire to be right, or do I see that you're also in pain, and reach out to you across that space that separates our hearts? Yoga is literally the realization that you're also suffering, and that if I can overcome my pride and reach out to you, I've just practiced samadhi. It sounds illogical, but the way to really win an argument is to be wrong!

This concept is reflected beautifully in the conflict resolution and therapeutic work of The Arbinger Institute:

> The more sure I am that I'm right, the more likely I will actually be mistaken. My need to be right makes it more likely that I will

be wrong! Likewise, the more sure I am that I am mistreated, the more likely I am to miss ways that I am mistreating others myself. My need for justification obscures the truth.[9]

This isn't about ignoring our own needs, or allowing ourselves to be abused. It's about reaching the apex of our humanity and seeing ourselves in others. To put it simply, being compassionate means respecting another person's feelings as well as my own. This is not to deny my feelings or subjugate myself to others, but to be strong enough to let the love back in. Let's be clear about this, because it's particularly important to understand the ways that our mutual awakening works. It's not that I'm doing you a favor by being compassionate to you. It's my own liberation that is at stake.

According to Rev. angel Kyodo williams:

> Once you are aware of how you are being policed, you can begin the process of self-liberating, from the position of realizing the mutuality of our liberation rather than suffering under the delusion that you are doing something for me. There is an intimacy in that realization. And because dharma is ultimately about accepting what is, it can undermine the need for control that keeps you invested in the policing of my body, thus freeing yours.[10]

Our liberation is tied together, whether you're abuser or abused, oppressor or oppressed. Working on yourself isn't about doing something for me; rather, as you become compassionate toward my needs, I help you undo some of your conditioning, and that in turn allows you to see more clearly. In a way, we are all constantly lifting each other up, over and over again, even if we don't see it, even if it doesn't feel like it.

## SAMADHI TODAY

Another way to see this is by flipping the script. Rather than thinking of my spiritual awakening as an individual achievement, I can think of my awakening as a way to love you. Your awakening is a way to love me. As only the great bhakti poet Hafiz could explain, "Your separation from God, from love, is the hardest work in this world."

A CUSHION FOR YOUR HEAD
Just sit there right now
Don't do a thing.
Just rest.

For your separation from God,
From love,

Is the hardest work
In this
World.

Let me bring you trays of food
And something
That you like to
Drink

You can use my soft words
As a cushion
For your
Head.[11]

That brings me back to the topic of reconsidering samadhi in these contemporary times. Michael Stone explains:

> With deep awakening, described by Patanjali as samadhi, there is an inherent understanding of the interconnected nature of reality. Again, samadhi literally means "integration." In samadhi we clearly see the nature of reality and live from that wisdom. However, no matter how cultivated our samadhi or how "big" our awakening, we still have to get along with others.[12]

I would even go a step further than Michael Stone and say that the true integration of samadhi means that our personal enlightenment is tied to the enlightenment of our community. In the end, community enlightenment is social justice and equity. I think it's fair to say that in this moment in time it is impossible to be enlightened without bringing your community along for the ride. Enlightenment is radical acceptance of life as it is, while simultaneously working to reduce the suffering of others.

Even in the *Hatha Yoga Pradipika*, the preeminent text on hatha yoga, we are told that we can only practice in a virtuous, well-ruled kingdom. That is not how I would describe the contemporary climate in the United States, or most of the world for that matter.

> One who practices hatha-yoga should live alone in a small monastery, situated a bow's length away from rocks, water, and fire, in a virtuous, well-ruled kingdom which is prosperous and free of disturbances.[13]

I think we could add to this list of preexisting conditions the health of the earth in general. If the earth itself is under siege, it isn't possible for an individual to find enlightenment. Our destiny is intimately connected to this planet and all the plants and animals that live here. If they are suffering, we are suffering. Our job is no longer to pursue freedom just for ourselves, but for all of us together.

## PRACTICING COMPASSION

So what do we do? How do we move toward samadhi in a time of inequity and in the midst of an environmental crisis? One way to think of the role of the individual in community enlightenment is service. Rather than working directly with the mind, service allows us to circumvent the mind with action. Service is a practice that asks us to engage in the world as a way of seeing ourselves more clearly. Service also includes taking care of our own body and mind—finding peace in our own life so that we don't burden others.

This is the meaning behind service and community care. It is a revolutionary idea because it goes against our capitalist training that tells us "every man for himself," and "may the best man win," as Amber Karnes previously explained. These ideas of individualism are ineffective and painful to ourselves and to the majority of humans. So why do they persist?

The great teacher and Vietnamese Buddhist monk Thich Nhat Hanh is such a powerful example of someone who transcends this limited sense of self and lives this vision of spirituality as social justice and interconnectedness. Because of his peace activism during the Vietnam War, he was exiled from Vietnam. He moved to France where he continued to teach—and practice—nonviolent activism, and was nominated for the Nobel Peace Prize in 1967 by Martin Luther King Jr., who said, "I do not personally know of anyone more worthy of [this prize] than this gentle monk from Vietnam. His ideas for peace, if applied, would build a monument to ecumenism, to world brotherhood, to humanity."[14]

Thich Nhat Hanh summarizes his revolutionary approach to spiritual activism in his poem, "Please Call Me by My True Names." In this reflection, he literally sees himself in others. I find this poem almost painful to read, but it represents a mind so expansive that it can see beyond right and wrong to the very essence of our humanity, to a compassion so deep that it cuts through selfishness and ego.

PLEASE CALL ME BY MY TRUE NAMES (song & poem)
Don't say that I will depart tomorrow—
even today I am still arriving.

Look deeply: every second I am arriving
to be a bud on a Spring branch,
to be a tiny bird, with still-fragile wings,
learning to sing in my new nest,
to be a caterpillar in the heart of a flower,
to be a jewel hiding itself in a stone.

I still arrive, in order to laugh and to cry,
to fear and to hope.

The rhythm of my heart is the birth and death
of all that is alive.

I am the mayfly metamorphosing
on the surface of the river.
And I am the bird
that swoops down to swallow the mayfly.

I am the frog swimming happily
in the clear water of a pond.
And I am the grass-snake
that silently feeds itself on the frog.

I am the child in Uganda, all skin and bones,
my legs as thin as bamboo sticks.
And I am the arms merchant,
selling deadly weapons to Uganda.

I am the twelve-year-old girl,
refugee on a small boat,
who throws herself into the ocean
after being raped by a sea pirate.
And I am the pirate,
my heart not yet capable
of seeing and loving.

I am a member of the politburo,
with plenty of power in my hands.
And I am the man who has to pay
his "debt of blood" to my people
dying slowly in a forced-labor camp.

My joy is like Spring, so warm
it makes flowers bloom all over the Earth.
My pain is like a river of tears,
so vast it fills the four oceans.

Please call me by my true names,
so I can hear all my cries and my laughter at once,
so I can see that my joy and pain are one.

Please call me by my true names,
so I can wake up,
and so the door of my heart

can be left open,
the door of compassion.[15]

Thich Nhat Hanh is asking us to step up, to evolve beyond simple ideas of right and wrong into a form of radical compassion. He's asking us for a true metamorphosis of our limited thinking into a mind that welcomes the experience of the other. What would that feel like? Is it possible that embracing our personal pain makes it easier to accept other people and their suffering? This is the opportunity of Thich Nhat Hanh's teaching, which he calls "interbeing," and it's reflected in the sharing (see sidebar) from Sarit Z. Rogers. She reflects on the process of othering—making some people less than, thereby dehumanizing them.

## EQUANIMITY BALANCES COMPASSION

How do you feel when you see someone crying or in pain? In many ways, the internal work you do processing your own personal feelings and past trauma dictates the depth of compassion you can have for others. Your personal practice becomes a training ground for your service in the world. It may dictate how present you can be. Many people think that spending time practicing yoga every day is selfish. But the truth is, the more you can process your own issues, the more effective you can be in the world, and the more compassion you can have for others.

I understand that being sensitive to other people's pain may feel pretty extreme when it's already overwhelming just trying to deal with your own suffering. So, your practice can also give you a sense of calm and equanimity, a moment of rest, which can create space for other people's pain. In her book *Real Change*, Sharon Salzberg explains, "Equanimity balances our caring so that compassionate action can be sustained and we won't drown under the weight of our sorrow."[16] This is such a useful teaching. If we become overwhelmed by the sorrow of the world—and it is overwhelming—we can easily get stuck in inaction and lethargy. The equanimity of yoga offers us enough space from the intensity of our feelings to have the energy to act.

The Gita says, "Equanimity of mind is yoga. Do everything, Arjuna, centered in that equanimity. Renouncing all attachments, you'll enjoy an

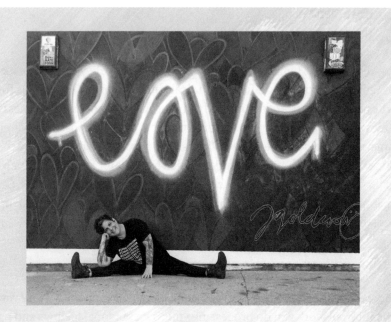

### SARIT Z. ROGERS

My yoga practice grounds me and nourishes me deeply, allowing for the expansion of my own capacity to hold space for and be a grounded presence and an empathetic witness to the populations I work with. Social justice and service/seva are what led me to teach. It has never been about the fancy space or the notoriety. Teaching and practicing yoga is bearing witness, humanizing the unseen in our society, dismantling systems of oppression, sharing compassion.

I remember the felt sense of making eye contact with an in-carcerated man at the county jail when I asked him his name—the name he wanted to be called, not his number or last name. He was in a solitary cage in the recreation room. There were tears in his eyes; a gentleness that emerged in his face when I said, "I see you." My practice allowed me to bear witness, to honor the feelings of my own powerlessness and also feel gratitude from this man as a result of being seen. My practice calls for justice and the impetus to ensure that difference is honored and not diminished by "otherness."

undisturbed mind in success or failure."[17] In other words, we'll avoid suffering by keeping an even, peaceful mind and not being attached to the results. This is easier said than done, and burnout in activists can easily occur when we don't see the results we were hoping for.

I know that after many years, I got tired of protesting in the streets. I couldn't see any direct positive results for those actions, even though I know they were valuable. My friends were still dying, my community was being ignored, and I was deeply frustrated. As Salzberg astutely described, I was drowning under the weight of my sorrow.

The way I avoided burnout was by looking to other activists for inspiration. In particular, I looked to young people, who are so often speaking truth to power. I remember the other young people who protested beside me in ACT UP and Queer Nation who inspired me for so many years. These days I'm inspired by young leaders like Malala, Isra Hirsi, Greta Thunberg and the Sunrise Movement, indigenous youth movements around the world, the Parkland students who organized against gun violence, and the young people who led Black Lives Matter protests in my small town. According to Malcolm X, "the young people are the ones who most quickly identify with the struggle and the necessity to eliminate the evil conditions that exist."[18]

Who inspires you? Can you think of someone who gives you energy to keep moving forward in your life, especially when life is challenging? Reflect on what it is about that person that is most inspirational to you. Consider how you can cultivate that quality in yourself.

## SEEING YOURSELF IN OTHERS

I also saw that my activism was my spiritual path. They weren't two different things. The more I studied and practiced yoga, the more I realized that compassion was the essence of the teachings. The Gita speaks of this eloquently. Krishna explains that the first goal on our path is realization of the spiritual truth within us and then to see that truth all around us—to see the same spirit everywhere and in everything. Then, Krishna explains, the next step is to literally feel the pleasure and pain of others as our own. This is the ultimate goal of yoga, according to the Gita.

The man equipped with yoga looks on all with an impartial eye, seeing Atman in all beings and all beings in Atman. He who sees Me everywhere and everything in Me, never vanishes from Me nor I from him.

The yogi who, anchored in unity, worships Me abiding in all beings lives and moves in Me, no matter how he lives and moves.

He who, by likening himself with others, senses pleasure and pain equally for all as for himself is deemed to be the highest yogi, O Arjuna.

This selection is from a translation of the Bhagavad Gita by Gandhi. Gandhi showed us how we could apply the yoga teaching directly to political and social justice struggles. But, Gandhi has become something of a controversial figure since he led efforts to overthrow the British colonial government in India, and there are reports that he supported a racist class system in South Africa when he lived there, as well as reports that he abused his wife.[19] I find it helpful to remember that Gandhi was the leader of a revolutionary movement that included an entire country, serving alongside many other inspiring leaders.

He offers a commentary after this section of the Gita, expounding on the ideas it brings to light:

He who acts towards others as if they were himself will meet their needs as if they were his own, will do to others what he would to himself, will learn to look upon himself and the world as one. He is a true yogi who is happy when others are happy and suffers when others suffer. Only that person who has reduced himself to a cipher, has completely shed his egotism, can claim to be so. He alone may be said to be such a person who has dedicated his all to God.[20]

Martin Buber, a Jewish theologian and philosopher from the early twentieth century, talked about how we can either relate to people as people—which he called "I-You,"—or we can relate to them as objects—which he called "I-It." To see people as objects means that we don't consider their feelings, or even their self-awareness, and instead focus on how they play into our narcissistic worldview.

At the heart of Buber's theology was his theory of dialogue—the idea that what matters is not understanding God in abstract, intellectual terms but, rather, entering into a relationship with him. Such a relationship, he believed, is possible only when we establish genuine relationships with one another. "Whoever goes forth to his You with his whole being and carries to it all the being of the world, finds him whom one cannot seek," he wrote. In daily life, we usually fail to live up to this ideal. We tend to treat the people and the world around us as things to be used for our benefit. Without this mind-set, which Buber called "I-It," there would be no science, economics, or politics. But, the more we engage in such thinking, the farther we drift from "I-You," his term for addressing other people directly as partners in dialogue and relationship. Only when we say "You" to the world do we perceive its miraculous strangeness and, at the same time, its potential for intimacy. Indeed, it's not only human beings who deserve to be called "You." As Buber wrote, even a cat or a piece of mica can summon up in us the feeling of a genuine encounter with another: "When something does emerge from among things, something living, and becomes a being for me . . . it is for me nothing but You!"[21]

As your practice creates windows into your mind, you may find that you tend to use the world and the people around you for your own benefit. But, when you see others as "You," as conscious beings, you become sensitive to their experience and realize that their suffering is as real as yours. This doesn't mean you become despondent and depressed about all the pain in the world, although sometimes that's a reasonable reaction.

## CONTENTMENT AS A PRACTICE

One of the most effective practices that is shared in the eight limbs of yoga is the teaching of santosha, which means "contentment." I was thinking about it the other morning as I woke up. I noticed myself going through a rapid series of thoughts and emotions. My first thought was a slight panic about the state of the world. Then, in the next moment, a very different thought came. As I lay in bed, I noticed how comfortable and warm I was.

I was overcome by a feeling of coziness and safety. I was filled with a sense of appreciation that flooded my body. I felt so lucky to have a warm bed, a safe place to sleep, and a roof over my head.

That was all in the first minute of being awake! Then I remembered a powerful meditation I once read by Thich Nhat Hanh, which he called, "The Un-Headache Meditation." In this meditation, he asks us to pause and recognize those moments when we are *not* in pain and *not* suffering, the times we don't have a headache. He asks us to appreciate those moments of feeling okay, and see that by focusing on them we can amplify their impact on our life. He explained that, "Sometimes your joy is the source of your smile, but sometimes your smile can be the source of your joy."

In the face of darkness and fear, it feels like bravery to smile, especially if it allows me to smile at my husband or someone on the street. It's not spiritual bypassing to try to focus on the little things that bring me joy or peace. Lifting myself up in this way is a big part of my practice. It's just as important as spending time exploring how I'm feeling and processing all of my emotions. Becoming conscious of my emotions is the heart of my practice, and therapy helps too! That way I can feel those moments when my frustration and my impatience arise and notice how I tend to take my feelings out on the people around me.

This is an essential service to myself and others—mostly because I'm not giving someone else a headache! When there is spaciousness, when I can bring my mind back to the safety of a warm bed, then I can offer support to my family, friends, students, and community. When I allow myself to smile, I can share the peace and also the pain of this journey. The smile becomes a gateway to sharing myself with the world.

> Can you spend a moment connecting with santosha, contentment? Consider what is going well in your life. What makes you smile?

Being at peace with myself, and experiencing contentment, gives my mind greater capacity to embrace other people's feelings and perspectives. In many ways, this is the goal of yoga: expanding our awareness to include multiple perspectives and a diversity of experiences—to expand our consciousness into a rainbow spectrum, a rainbow mind.

Rainbows are a glimpse into another dimension. They allow us to see beautiful colors when there is usually only white light. Red, orange, yellow, green, blue, indigo, violet; rainbows represent the entire spectrum of visible light, an analogy for the spectrum of human experience. We are all unique, even though we share the same essence. This is the symbolism of the rainbow flag that is used to represent the queer community.

> What I liked about the rainbow is that it fits all of us.
> It's all the colors.
> It represents all the genders.
> It represents all the races.
> It's the rainbow of humanity.
> —GILBERT BAKER, CREATOR OF THE RAINBOW FLAG

My goal is to open my mind to the diversity of experience, even going beyond the human to embrace the experience of animals and the earth itself. I seek to live in alignment with that awareness instead of hiding in my ego-mind's silo of self-righteousness. In this expansive place I am most alive and most open. I am completely full.

This reminds me of one of the Shanti mantras from the *Brihadaranyaka Upanishad* (5.1.1) which speaks to the fullness of creation and describes a state of mind, beyond ego, that is big enough to embrace that fullness. It's a paradoxical state that we may have trouble comprehending on an intellectual level: The more I give, the more I have. This fullness comes from that fullness, yet that fullness remains forever full. The more I love, the more love I have.

> *om purnam adah purnam idam*
> *purnat purnam udachyate*
> *purnasya purnamadaya*
> *purnamevavashishyate*
> *om shanti, shanti, shanti*

> That is full this also is full.
> This Fullness came from that Fullness.
> Though this Fullness came from that Fullness
> That Fullness remains forever full.
> Om peace, peace, peace[22]

# 6 | HONEST REFLECTION

YOGA IS FREE. Okay, you probably had to pay for this book, so I guess it doesn't feel free. But this book isn't yoga. Yoga can't be bought or sold. These are universal spiritual teachings that have existed for thousands of years. I find it useful to remember that yoga is unchanging even though the vehicles we're learning it through are always changing.

This book is a reflection on some of the ways that yoga has shaped me. I hope some of this is useful to you so that you can allow yoga to mold you and fold you into unusual shapes, give you a different perspective, and take you to new places within yourself. I'm amazed at where yoga has taken me. The past fifteen years or so I've had the privilege of traveling around the world teaching. I've been able to visit amazing places and get to know them through their local yoga teachers, which has been the thrill of a lifetime.

More than just traveling to amazing locations, yoga has taken me to places in myself that I wouldn't have known how to find otherwise, places that I thought I had lost. Yoga is like the secret door inside the wardrobe. Every time I practice I seem to go somewhere away from my daily worries and stress. And that's huge, because so often I feel trapped in my own mind and in my own life. As Amina Naru describes in her sharing, yoga can help excavate internal space by allowing us a way to work with our own psychological debris and giving us a way to process personal trauma.

## ANXIETY

I've been using yoga to help me handle mild anxiety for my entire adult life, and it has been incredibly effective. But three years ago, just a few months after my mother's death, I had a severe anxiety attack. I ended up in the emergency room since I didn't know what was happening to me.

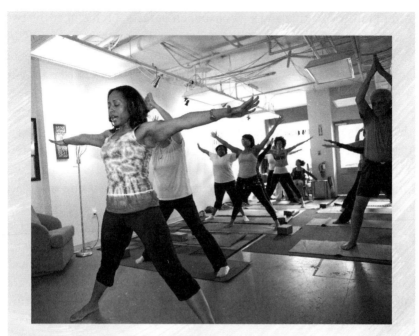

## AMINA NARU

My yoga practice has excavated internal space and knowledge that has allowed me to show up for others who have suffered and live with adverse patterns and behaviors as the result of trauma. The work started with myself first and my own demons. The practices of yoga began to peel back the layers of emotional, physical, and psychological debris that were haunting my relationships and stunting spiritual growth. Once I was able to see my own struggles, resistances, and patterns, I was able to do the work in my life off of the mat. I discovered a deep well of passion to serve and compassion for people as my rigid and limited mental programming became more flexible and expansive with empathy, understanding, patience, and oneness. It is from this well and my self-care practices I am continually supported in my work for humanity.

After hours of waiting and a whole bunch of tests, I remember the two emergency room doctors coming to talk to me. The one in charge said, "We can't find any physical cause for your symptoms, and we think it might be an anxiety attack." I laughed out loud and said, "That can't be right. I'm a yoga teacher!"

For the longest time after that, I couldn't bring myself to accept the fact that I have severe anxiety. I had kept up a regular yoga and meditation practice for thirty years, and I spent time every day calming my nervous system and working with my mind. But I couldn't deny what had happened. For a while, my practice became very difficult. What had once been a sanctuary started to feel like an alien world.

I know that yoga has been proven to support people with anxiety,[1] but it took me a while to find my way back to a formal practice. Looking back, I can see that one positive outcome is that my experience gave me so much compassion for the resistance I had seen in my students over the years. All of a sudden, I completely understood how difficult it could be to turn within, and why the subtle practices of pranayama (breathing practices) and meditation are particularly challenging. I was a beginner again.

Luckily, I haven't had another anxiety attack like that one, although the fear still lingers. Since then, my practice has evolved in so many ways. Most of all, I've let go of the striving that came out of wanting to be a "good" yoga student. Now, I spend time every day with myself, but not always in the kind of formal practice that I used to require of myself. I move and find stillness in more spontaneous ways that support my mental and physical health in the moment. Sometimes I dance around the room and sometimes I lift weights and then do some asana and relaxation.

One of the things that helped me with my anxiety was the support of an amazing yoga therapist who allowed me to be a student again. I had fallen into a trap that is so common for teachers: we forget to keep learning. We think we know enough and stop there. I'm not going to go as far as to say that I'm grateful for my anxiety, because that is clichéd nonsense. I've tried to engage with my anxiety to expand the way I conceive of, and relate to, my own mind. I accept that fear, worry—and even panic—are normal parts of my humanity. I don't need to run away from those painful feelings toward some mystical idea of peace, which is what I was doing before.

## EMBRACING FAILURE

Honestly, a bigger problem was that having anxiety made me feel like a failure as a yoga practitioner and teacher. How could I have anxiety if the focus of my life has been learning to calm my nervous system and control my mind? Well, I think the answer lies in the latter part of that statement: controlling the mind is a dangerous game. Since my anxiety attack, I've been exploring new ways to approach my mind with kindness, and a new understanding of what I need. Instead of controlling my mind, I'm working on repairing my relationship with myself. Kabir describes it well:

THE FAILURE
I talk to my inner lover, and I say, why such rush?
We sense that there is some sort of spirit that loves birds and
    animals and the ants—
perhaps the same one who gave a radiance to you in your
    mother's womb.
Is it logical you would be walking around entirely orphaned now?
The truth is you turned away yourself,
and decided to go into the dark alone.
Now you are tangled up in others, and have forgotten what you
    once knew,
and that's why everything you do has some weird failure in it.[2]

I love Kabir's premise that, "you turned away yourself . . . and that's why everything you do has some weird failure in it " He gets right to the heart of the issue of identifying with ego-mind instead of spirit. I also love the idea of normalizing failure. Isn't that what it means to be human? Isn't life a succession of failures that we learn from? How can you learn if you don't fail?

Failure is the direct outcome of practice. Failure is what we get to do every time we get on the mat. We get to fail at this pose or that pose. We get to fail at relaxing when we lie in Shavasana and our nervous system is buzzing with caffeine, and we get to fail at meditating every time our mind wanders. I've never practiced yoga and not failed, and that's exactly the point.

Failure is the key to yoga. It's like that expression, "the broken place is where the light shines through." The failure is where the light of yoga shines through to expose our most tender places—our wounds. It illuminates the limits of the body and mind, not so we can overcome them through sheer force, but so we can love them more. How else can we become whole (healed) without completely embracing our mistakes and our failures?

If we don't accept failure, we live in an imaginary bubble of our ego-centered imagination. We deny anything that goes against our self-image; we create "alternate truths." The first step in social justice and equity work is identifying our shortcomings. We need to admit to our prejudices, our unconscious bias, and our mistakes. We need to clearly see our failures so we can do better. But how can we see them if we are constantly defending ourselves, no matter how many mistakes we make and how many people we harm?

We can learn how to fail in public by apologizing for our mistakes. If I make a social media post that is offensive or incorrect, I can either defend my position over and over in angry comments, or I can say, "I was wrong, and I'm sorry." As Maya Angelou famously said, "I did then what I knew how to do. Now that I know better, I do better."[3] There is tremendous wisdom in that simple statement.

Yes, yoga practice is a journey to self-love, but not in an egotistical way. This is where we so often get it wrong. It's about loving our differences instead of hiding them, celebrating our limitations instead of denying them, and literally investing in our failures. By embracing failure, we integrate our humanity and our spirituality. Rather than dance between them, we can love our limited human body and mind as fascinating expressions of our spirit, and appreciate how essential they are to our journey.

Failure reminds us that complete identification with the body-mind is unhealthy, and that we haven't been "orphaned" here, as Kabir describes. Our spirit isn't separate from this human experience, rather it's the glue holding it all together. There is no part of us that is not connected to spirit, even the ugly, dirty, and painful parts. And the way to experience spirit isn't by denying the ugly parts, but by loving the most orphaned parts of ourselves more.

Can you think of an experience in your life that felt like a failure, but in the end was actually a kind of success?

## COURAGE TO FACE YOURSELF

I've found that my anxiety has many triggers, but the greatest one is fear. The Gita talks directly about how yoga removes fear. Krishna explains to Arjuna, "On this path no effort is wasted, nor is there any danger of adverse effects. Even a little practice of this yoga protects one from great fear."[4] Protecting us from fear can also be understood as giving us courage, and courage to face ourselves is one of the powerful benefits of yoga.

Fear is a sign of ego. It's that concept of a separate individual self that we're working to see more clearly in our yoga practice. We don't need to squash the ego; we just need to see it for what it is. Our fear is actually exposing that part of ourselves to the light of day. It's exposing our most sensitive places, the parts of ourselves we cover up and deny. Fear is a gateway to understanding our ego. Of course, *ego* is a confusing word to use because it has different meanings in yoga and psychology.

Generally, ego in yoga represents the separate self that we want to overcome, but in psychology it's an essential element of our personality. Maybe we can learn from that definition? The real question is, can you embrace that scared, small part of yourself, or do you judge it and hide it away? This is the challenge of a spiritual practice, and it speaks to the way our practice can either heal or exacerbate our underlying issues. We can see the state of our ego in the quality of our inner dialogue. The way we talk to ourselves says a lot about whether the ego is an integrated part of our being or if we're at war with ourselves.

One example of this is my lifelong struggle with shyness. I was extremely shy when I was younger, and honestly, I still am even though I speak in front of people all the time. My practice has helped me overcome what is really a type of egoism. My shyness was based on a fragile ego that was overly concerned with what other people think of me. In many ways, it was connected to being gay and being in the closet. It was only when I began to let go of my attachment to other people's opinions of me that I could feel freer.

What does your internal dialogue sound like? Do you speak to yourself with anger or with kindness?

## COMING OUT

Do you ever find yourself clenching your jaw waiting for something bad to happen? Or waking up in the morning with a feeling of dread? These feelings can be traced back to fear, whether they come in small doses or huge heart-stopping moments of panic. One particularly fearful time that stands out in my life was when I came out of the closet and told my mother I was gay. I was seventeen and confused. I found myself living a secret life and not sharing it with her. Speaking my truth that day was a major victory, and it made me understand a little about the way fear ruled my life.

Those of us who are marginalized often internalize our oppression as fear, and I was very afraid. I was afraid to be different and to be excluded from society—tossed out like garbage. It wasn't until I practiced yoga regularly that I was able to recognize my emotions and realize that I was living in a constant state of fear, with a mild panic just under the surface.

It was Shavasana that gave me away. I remember getting very quiet, maybe for the first time ever without alcohol or drugs, and I jerked awake like I had fallen asleep too quickly. But I hadn't fallen asleep. My nervous system was reacting to its first opportunity to unwind the tension it had been storing up for years. That tension had served a purpose to protect me. It saved my life by giving me quick reflexes to duck out of the way when some drunk man threw a beer bottle at my head and yelled, "Queer!" But the tension was also slowly killing me with stress and anxiety.

Soon yoga became my refuge, and I was able to undo a lot of the hidden tension in my body. I also realized that so many people carry similar burdens: knots of anxiety in our jaws and necks. As I started to teach yoga, by sharing it with the HIV/AIDS community in the late nineties, I saw the power of yoga to offer relief from the fear that silently engulfed us.

In our shared suffering I also saw the possibility of salvation. The strength of a group OM echoed in my heart louder than when I chanted it alone. In yoga, I found the possibility of overcoming fear through community. Those of us who look different, move different, love different—we needed to support each other and hold each other in a strong embrace.

## WHEN I TURN WITHIN I FIND YOU THERE

Yoga offered me a way to connect with others. It's a paradox: when I turn within I find you there. It is in the presence of community that I can release my fear. I feel carried and cared for. I feel like I have a special place in the world, and that I belong.

That is why I decided to start teaching yoga in 1995. I had been studying for many years at that point, but it occurred to me that I could put my energy into serving my community and sharing yoga. I decided to create special classes for people with HIV and AIDS. After I got certified, I immediately created classes at the hospital closest to the Castro in San Francisco, which is the hub of the gay community.

In those classes, we would always start with a check-in or discussion and then do a full yoga practice. These were two-hour sessions that met multiple times a week for close to fifteen years. The regularity and consistency of these classes are the way we built a community and got to know each other. It was also a chance for me to share some of the teachings in more depth than a traditional yoga class format would allow. We would usually read from the Gita or the Yoga Sutras. Actually, over those years we must have read through the entirety of those texts at least three or four times each.

So many incredible people participated in those classes, and they all had such a strong influence on my understanding of the teachings and the way I share them. I remember one longtime student named John. He was in his mid-twenties, had AIDS, and was really depressed. He came to the classes on and off for a few years, and I would always worry when I didn't see him for a while. He shared with us that he was an alcoholic and that he was using alcohol to deal with his depression and fear of dying.

In those days, AIDS treatments were still mostly ineffective, and John knew he was dying. John and I were about the same age, and it was hard for me to give him any advice or to question his choices. I had to ask myself what I would be doing if I were dying of AIDS. Drinking away his worries seemed like an understandable reaction.

But the whole group was deeply concerned for him. I remember one day John came to class after being absent for a few weeks. He walked in and quickly apologized for being gone so long. The reaction from the whole group was powerful. He was met with joy and love. He was hugged and his presence was celebrated. No one was judging him, simply appreciating the fact that he made it there that day. I remember some other students in the group offering support, reaching out to talk after class, and asking him if he was okay. Then John stopped coming, and we never heard from him again. We found out that he had died, and we were all devastated. We talked about feeling like we wished we could have done more for John, but we were all glad we had offered moments of peace and comfort to him.

There was such power in that community. We were holding each other and ourselves in a way that felt loving and kind. The bond we formed may have grown out of desperation, but it transformed into a powerful connection. Over the years, we began to invite people with other disabilities into the group, and a number of the students went on to become yoga teachers themselves. In fact, that core group was the beginning of what eventually became the nonprofit, Accessible Yoga.

> What supports your spiritual practices? Do you enjoy practicing in a group or by yourself? Do you enjoy having a regular routine or being more creative?

# 7 | DEATH IS THE ULTIMATE TEACHER

MY MOTHER DIED over three years ago, and my father died just last year. Ever since their deaths, I find myself spending a lot of time thinking about my own death. It has somehow lifted the veil on my own mortality. It also reminds me of at least a dozen close friends and students who died from AIDS when I was in my twenties. If I spend some time thinking about it, I'm sure I could think of twice as many people who died back then.

I remember feeling stuck, and I didn't know how to make sense of so much sickness and death. I was also heartbroken and filled with questions. Mostly, I didn't know how to move forward with my life when death was so present. I realized that all I could do was explore the burning question of spirituality: Does part of us live on when we die?

Isn't that what we're all wondering? Don't we all think about what happens when we die? Do we fall asleep and never wake, as our body returns back to its earthly home? Or, does a spark within us travel on to some other place? Maybe we're reincarnated into another life—as a newborn baby, an ant, a dog, or a plant. Perhaps our spirit merges with a larger communal spirit, and we experience some kind of oneness. Maybe you believe your spirit goes on to heaven or hell. Personally, I was obsessed with these questions, and I dove into the yoga teachings to try to find answers.

One clear answer came in the Yoga Sutras, where Patanjali lists the five obstacles to our enlightenment. They are all based on ignorance of our true nature, avidya. The last obstacle is *abhinivesha*, fear of death, which is also an attachment, or clinging, to life. He explains, "Clinging to life, flowing by its own potency [due to past experience], exists even in the wise."[1] I saw that yoga is preparation for death. Why else would we end every practice with Shavasana, Corpse Pose? Yoga is helping us find the right relationship with our body—and its limitations. I began to find what I was looking for, but studying the Bhagavad Gita was even more revealing.

## THE DESPONDENCY OF ARJUNA

In one of the most respected translations of the Gita, Eknath Easwaran introduces the scripture with an explanation of the necessity of applying these teachings directly to our lives. He explains that the Gita offers more than an incredible story or esoteric philosophy. It offers down-to-earth lessons on living spirituality gifted to us from ages of experience and wisdom. The Gita is a part of the ancient epic, the Mahabharata, and it was written by the sage Vyasa.

> Scholars can debate the point forever, but when the Gita is practiced, I think, it becomes clear that the struggle the Gita is concerned with is the struggle for self-mastery. It was Vyasa's genius to take the whole great Mahabharata epic and see it as metaphor for the perennial war between the forces of light and the forces of darkness in every human heart. Arjuna and Krishna are then no longer merely characters in a literary masterpiece. Arjuna becomes Everyman, asking the Lord himself, Sri Krishna, the perennial questions about life and death—not as a philosopher, but as the quintessential man of action. Thus read, the Gita is not an external dialogue but an internal one: between the ordinary human personality, full of questions about the meaning of life, and our deepest Self, which is divine.
>
> There is, in fact, no other way to read the Gita and grasp it as spiritual instruction. If I could offer only one key to understanding this divine dialogue, it would be to remember that it takes place in the depths of consciousness and that Krishna is not some external being, human or superhuman, but the spark of divinity that lies at the core of the human personality. This is not literary or philosophical conjecture; Krishna says as much to Arjuna over and over: "I am the Self in the heart of every creature, Arjuna, and the beginning, middle, and end of their existence."[2]

In the opening of the Gita, Arjuna faces a terrible conundrum: Should he fight his extended family in a justified war? The other side, the Kauravas, who are relatives of Arjuna, have destroyed the kingdom with their selfishness and immorality. He and his brothers, the Pandavas, tried to negotiate with them, but the Kauravas continually trick them and cheat them. The Pandavas were tricked into agreeing to be banished for twelve years under the premise that when they returned the kingdom would be restored to them. But once they returned they were forced to continue their exile for another twelve years. In the meantime, the kingdom was being destroyed by the Kauravas' greed and evil.

As the Gita begins, Arjuna is on the battlefield in his chariot with Krishna as his charioteer. He instructs Krishna to bring his chariot into the middle of the field so he can see who he's up against: the Kauravas and Krishna's million-strong army. Arjuna is overcome with emotion. Trembling, and with his mind whirling, he tells Krishna all the reasons why he shouldn't fight this war. He explains that he's not interested in winning, he doesn't want to fight his cousins, and he doesn't want to destroy society by killing families. These concerns are important if we consider the Gita's narrative and the idea of a just war. But if we consider the Gita as an analogy for an inner spiritual battle, these concerns take on a different light. In that light, they remind me of all the attachments in my mind: the things I think I'm giving up when I invest in spirit rather than in worldly experience.

Arjuna's concerns also remind me of the kind of logic my mind comes up with when I see suffering or evil in the world and I don't act. I'm not proud to admit it, but there are so many times when I know I could speak up or act but I don't. After arguing with Krishna, Arjuna finally drops his bow and arrow, collapses in utter despair, and says:

> In the dark night of my soul I feel desolation. In my self-pity I see not the way of righteousness. I am thy disciple, come to thee in supplication: be a light unto me on the path of my duty. For neither the kingdom of the earth, nor the kingdom of the gods in heaven, could give me peace from the fire of sorrow which thus burns my life.[3]

Think of a time when you could have acted or spoken up against harm of some kind, and consider why you didn't. Maybe you walked by a homeless person asking for help or didn't attend a demonstration for a cause you believe it. Or maybe you heard a homophobic or racist comment at work and didn't say anything. What was it that kept you from acting or speaking? Try not to beat yourself up about it, but consider it in a neutral way. Try to find the root of that inaction.

## TRUE SURRENDER

This moment, when Arjuna surrenders to Krishna, is the turning point in the Gita. Arjuna represents our ego-mind, and this is when we see Arjuna admit that he may not have all the answers. It's that moment when we collapse in anguish and realize that all the worldly accomplishments and success we're seeking won't change the fact that we can't take it with us in the end. It's a realization that we tend to avoid at all costs, but it is literally the moment we begin to open our eyes in our spiritual awakening.

I mentioned earlier that yoga practice begins when we lie sobbing on our yoga mats, not when we perform a perfect Trikonasana. This is what I was referring to. The pain and sorrow we feel are actually the result of releasing years of shoring up the ego-mind with false attachments and beliefs. These moments offer the purest potential for our growth, but we can't seek them out. Our intellect wants to control the process, make it work on our timeline, and decide when and how much we are willing to surrender. But it doesn't work that way. Surrender is the blossoming of a flower within us. You can't pull the petals of the bud open to make the flower bloom faster. The bud has its own wisdom, and so do our hearts.

I often wonder about the way plants experience time. We can see that they grow, bloom, and die. But we don't see it happening in real time. Plant time doesn't unfold in the same way that we experience time. Spirit also has its own timeline, regardless of what we want or expect. The point is, we need to be patient with ourselves. A regular practice can help to support our spiritual growth, but the awakening we seek may not come when we want it to.

Remember, this surrender is not to someone or something outside of ourselves—not to a teacher or guru. Arjuna surrenders to Krishna, who represents his own true self. It's a surrender of the false sense of self to the part of ourselves that is unchanging, immortal, and everlasting. It's a recognition of the truth that yoga seeks to impart: we are spiritual beings masquerading as mortal beings.

The Gita's teaching is a reflection of the *Katha Upanishad*, especially Nichiketas's dialogue with Death:

Death: There is the path of joy, and there is the path of pleasure. Both attract the soul. Who follows the first comes to good; who follows pleasure reaches not the end.

The two paths lie in front of man. Pondering on them, the wise man chooses the path of joy; the fool takes the path of pleasure. . . .

When the wise rests his mind in contemplation on our God beyond time, who invisibly dwells in the mystery of things and in the heart of man, then he rises above pleasure and sorrow.

When a man has heard and has understood and, finding the essence, reaches the Inmost, then he finds joy in the Source of joy.[4]

I find it useful to contemplate the difference between pleasure and joy. It's not that pleasure isn't essential, but it seems dependent on external factors and it's so often the focus of my mental chatter. On the other hand, I find that joy arises from within when I feel at peace or when my life feels like it's in alignment—when I surrender.

## YOU DO NOT DIE WHEN THE BODY DIES

After Arjuna surrenders, Krishna smiles and begins to teach him about yoga. I love the idea of Krishna smiling with the patient wisdom of an experienced teacher or friend. He smiles knowing that everything will be okay. Krishna then begins his instruction in yoga with a key lesson about the immortality of the spirit. In one of the most well-known verses in the Gita, he explains:

You were never born; you will never die. You have never changed; you can never change. Unborn, eternal, immutable, immemorial, you do not die when the body dies.[5]

It's a message I can't hear enough times, and was especially so when I was dealing with my mother's impending death. As my mother got very sick, I kept thinking that I needed to talk to her about death and how she felt about dying. I had this idea that talking it through would somehow make it easier for her, and for me. So, a number of times, I tried to broach the subject with her. Each time, she would either ignore me or quickly change the subject. I eventually gave up, concluding that she wasn't ready to talk about her impending death and that she was in denial about it.

As she got weaker it became harder for her to speak, and for the last few weeks she could barely open her eyes. I thought I had lost my chance to help her process her feelings about dying. But I began to notice something amazing. Every time someone she loved was near her, she would struggle to open her eyes and summon just enough energy to say, "I love you. I love you so much." This became a mantra for her in those final days: "I love you. I love you so much," whispered through dry lips over and over.

One day, my kids came with me to see her for what would be their final visit with their grandmother. I could see her struggling to wake up for them, and I heard her tell them how much she loved them with so much conviction that it made me cry. In that moment, it dawned on me that she was answering all my questions about death. Rather than have an intellectual conversation with me about it, she was teaching me that love is the answer to all the questions, and that loving is the purpose of life.

I know my mother's love is still with me even though she is gone, but sometimes I forget and feel lost. So now, I'm trying to find ways to unearth that love for myself, in a process that can be surprisingly hard. I realize that some people never had a loving parent and may be used to that struggle, but for me it's still new.

I also know that the ultimate purpose of yoga and meditation is to feel love. I can use my time in meditation to examine where I've gotten caught up in the world. It's amazing how confused my ego-mind gets—convincing me that love will come from outside of me when I get something or accomplish something. It's only through practice that I can remind myself it's safe to *be* love instead of constantly trying to *get* love.

Sit comfortably, and notice the breath without changing it. Bring to mind someone that you love. It can be someone who has died or is no longer in your life. Try to picture them clearly in your mind's eye. Begin to notice how you feel when you think of them. In your mind say, "I love you" a few times. If your mind wanders, just notice it and then come back to their image and say, "I love you." After a few minutes sit quietly and notice how you feel.

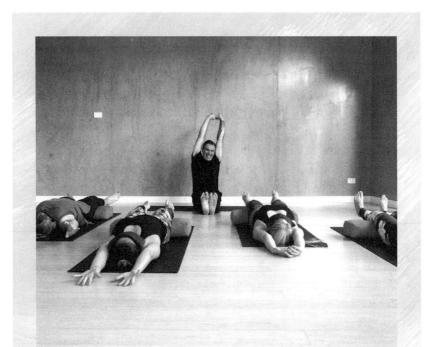

### RANE BOWEN

My stomach was removed around five years ago due to stomach cancer, and I find that I hold a lot of tension in the area where my stomach used to be. In my yoga practice I'm able to recognize this fact, soften, and sit with it. Facing death made me really sit with the questions of what is important in this life. Taking action to help make this world a better place is one of the answers that came through.

Our love of yoga inspired me and my wife, Jo, to start the Flow Artists Podcast, which has been a connecting thread between us and some incredible activists, artists, and authors who also practice yoga. Sharing their work with the world is both an act of service but also enriching for us as humans, encouraging us to question and look within, just as we do on the mat.

## GRIEF

The COVID-19 pandemic has reminded us of the reality of death in the midst of our lives. The death of so many has thrown into stark relief lessons about the importance of love. In a reflection on mortality in the face of the pandemic, hospice doctor BJ Miller describes it this way:

> Beyond fear and isolation, maybe this is what the pandemic holds for us: the understanding that living in the face of death can set off a cascade of realization and appreciation. Death is the force that shows you what you love and urges you to revel in that love while the clock ticks. Reveling in love is one sure way to see through and beyond yourself to the wider world, where immortality lives. A pretty brilliant system, really, showing you who you are (limited) and all that you're a part of (vast). As a connecting force, love makes a person much more resistant to obliteration.[6]

In my heart, I know that death is the greatest teacher, but sometimes I'm not a very good student. I need to be taught some lessons over and over again. I notice this with painful emotions. I know I need to embrace the pain of my grief, anger, and fear in order to process it in a healthy way, but it's something I'd still rather avoid. All those emotions usually merge into anxiety when I ignore them. Eventually my anxiety feels like a geyser of pain that I keep trying to cover over, but it keeps seeping out. Releasing those feelings can feel overwhelming, but it's usually the healthiest way forward—if I'm ready.

Lama Rod Owens explores the power of grieving:

> When we are touching into the hurt, the hurt begins to inform us. When we actually begin to mourn and grieve, that mourning helps us to experience a spaciousness within our experience. The hurt isn't the central thing anymore; it's something that's happening within the spaciousness of other things that can arise. I grieve every day. When I give the mourning lots of space, the anger has lots of space. The anger is like, "Thank you, finally, for taking care of the hurt." The energy of anger is still there. If I am grieving, then I

can actually channel the energy of anger, not into trying to protect myself, not into trying to hurt other people, but rechannel it into benefiting others.[7]

An effective yoga practice is designed to create space for us to process our feelings, since unprocessed emotions are actually pulling the mind here and there. When we're practicing, the mind is pulled back into the present moment, giving us an opportunity to notice how we feel right now. When I notice myself avoiding a strong feeling, I try to stop and have an honest talk with myself. Often the feelings are connected to some pain that I've felt or avoided trying to feel. I usually have to get on my mat and do some asanas before I can begin to experience deep emotions. The movement gets energy moving in my body, and emotions are a form of energy.

Most of the time, when an emotion comes, it's usually grief. Grief over what I've lost or what has changed, accompanied by the feeling that time is fleeting, and that everyone I love will eventually die—or I will. When I explore it more deeply it seems like grief is simply love that no longer has an outlet. It's pent up, frustrated love that feels hopeless and lost.

I'm sure it sounds very depressing, but I think it's good to be totally honest with myself once in a while. That honesty (satya) is the key to living in the truth. The truth is that I am a spiritual being, and my essence is immortal. This represents a seismic shift that changes how I feel about myself and my life. This shift in thinking is the message of the Gita, and is described powerfully in this passage where Krishna instructs Arjuna in the nature of birth and death:

> You speak sincerely, but your sorrow has no cause. The wise grieve neither for the living nor for the dead. There has never been a time when you and I and the kings gathered here have not existed, nor will there be a time when we will cease to exist. As the same person inhabits the body through childhood, youth, and old age, so too at the time of death he attains another body. The wise are not deluded by these changes.
>
> The impermanent has no reality; reality lies in the eternal. Those who have seen the boundary between these two have

attained the end of all knowledge. Realize that which pervades the universal and is indestructible; no power can affect this unchanging, imperishable reality. The body is mortal, but that which dwells in the body is immortal and immeasurable. Therefore, Arjuna, fight in this battle.[8]

## DEATH ISN'T A FAILURE

Contemporary yoga practice reinforces many of the myths of the capitalist system that it's evolving within. In order for yoga to be our sanctuary, we have to make sure we aren't using it to oppress ourselves. Yoga is essentially a spiritual practice, connecting us firmly with that essence, which is called *atman* or *purusha* in Sanskrit. In modern postural yoga, we have focused on some kind of optimum physical ability, or "wellness," as the goal of the practice, which is itself often at odds with the spiritual teachings.

Yoga reminds us that we're not just the body-mind: we are eternal. When we obsess over making complicated shapes with the body we may be missing out on these larger goals. I also worry that modern yoga teaches us to value health in a way that reinforces ableist ideals of nondisabled bodies being morally superior to ill, old, or disabled bodies. When we release this judgmental attitude that certain bodies are superior to others and that one way of being in a body is better than other ways, then we can connect more directly to the goals of the practice.

Another way to think of it is to consider the way that the teachings approach death. There is a clear message in the teachings that we can overcome death through yoga, but that's not what we think it means. Overcoming death in the teachings isn't about keeping the body alive forever. It's about identifying with the part of us that never dies. That's a very different goal for our yoga practice. We're not in a battle with time to retain some ideal of perfect health. We're in a battle to clearly see the ego-mind for what it is and to begin identifying with spirit instead.

> If the goal of yoga is wellness or healing on a completely physical level, then are illness, disability, and especially death, a failure? How can death be a failure when it is the one thing that is absolutely guaranteed in life?

This fight against death is so ingrained in us that we have a hard time recognizing the way it impacts our self-image and the way we think of other people who are sick or dying. When we embrace illness and death as an intimate part of life it can free up a lot of space in our minds, and free us from ignorance. We can begin to see more clearly the emotional attachment we have to our body and to the bodies of the people we love. This attachment is very real. It's like a cloud of grief that follows us around and that we pretend isn't there. Focusing on our grief, and learning how to process it, is a very different and necessary practice than pursuing optimum health at any cost.

The way we respond to grief, or don't, reminds me of Patanjali's basic teaching. In his opening statement he declares, *yogash chitta vritti nirodhah*, "stillness of the mind is yoga." Here, the term *vritti* is used to describe thoughts, or disturbances of the mind. Personally, I find that emotions disturb my mind more than any other thoughts. Perhaps a completely new way to approach that sutra could be, "Yoga is learning how to process emotion in a healthy way that allows us to experience freedom."

Processing emotions in a healthy way is a balancing act. Some people feel that they are overly emotional, and many people are experiencing the effects of long-term or short-term trauma. This is important to keep in mind as we build our practice and seek the appropriate tools to support the healthy processing of emotions. Each of us needs a slightly different combination of support to help us come back to neutral when we feel overcome by emotions.

That process is called nervous-system regulation, and it can be one of the most powerful elements of yoga practice. In particular, breathing practices, relaxation, chanting, and meditation are very effective at regulating the nervous system. They allow us an opportunity to come back to neutral if we have been triggered in some way. But it only works if the practice is appropriate for that person in that moment. In the end, yoga offers us tools to handle big feelings in a healthy way, but each of us has to find our own individual combination of practices.

Remember, most of us need support to process emotions, past trauma, or challenging times in our lives. It can be psychotherapy, yoga therapy, or some form of practice to specifically deal with our emotions. While I think yoga can help us handle our emotional life, I also feel strongly that it's not enough. Often a combination of emotional support, medication, and yoga may be needed to help us get through challenging times. There is no shame in needing support: even Arjuna, the greatest warrior in the land, desperately needed the support of Krishna to resolve his grief and step forward into his life.

# SUMMARY OF PART ONE

IN THE FIRST SECTION of the book, I've tried to offer a slightly different perspective on some of the most essential yoga teachings. I'm interested in finding a useful and effective interpretation of yoga philosophy that can guide us in our lives. The fact is, these teachings have survived for thousands of years because they are so applicable and user-friendly. These ancient yoga teachings aren't meant to just be studied academically, they are meant to be lived in the here and now.

Yoga asks us to identify with our unchanging essence, our spirit, rather than with the constantly changing body and mind. This seemingly simple idea can create a major shift in our lives, and in our experience of life. This idea, of moving from impermanent to permanent, is the definition of spirituality.

Spirituality isn't just something we find through religion. It's a way of perceiving ourselves and the world around us. It's the knowledge that truth rests in my heart as well as in yours. Regardless of circumstance or background, we share this same essence. The diversity of creation—including every single human—can be embraced rather than feared. With practice, we can begin to see the unity of life in the diversity of its manifestation.

I shared my personal stories of fear and anxiety to explore the ways that we can find the truths of yoga in our darkest days. Death and grief have the ability to make the most important parts of life stand out in stark relief. What is left when we die? What is left of the people we've lost?

In the end, the question of yoga is whether we can listen to the advice of our ancient teachers and cultivate clear perception. Can we learn from the pain and suffering in our own lives to show us a different way forward? Suffering offers opportunities for course correcting. Rather than allowing ourselves to continue to be motivated by selfishness and egoism, suffering is there to crack our heart open, create greater self-awareness, and ignite compassion for ourselves and others.

# PART TWO

# OUTER REVOLUTION

Helping, fixing, and serving represent three different ways of seeing life. When you help, you see life as weak. When you fix, you see life as broken. When you serve, you see life as whole. Fixing and helping may be the work of the ego, and service the work of the soul.

—RACHEL NAOMI REMEN

# 8 | YOGA IS SERVICE

THE SECOND SECTION of this book is focused on how we put these teachings into practice. I'm interested in how we can engage the teachings in resolving conflict within ourselves, and also in the world at large. This is one of the incredible things about yoga: the work we do on ourselves has a direct correlation to the way we affect the world around us. I'm not offering a specific form for your work in the world; of course, that's up to you. But by building courage and compassion through our practice, we can move out into the world in an openhearted way and make social justice a central part of our practice. This is the same message that Krishna shares with Arjuna in the Gita:

> The ignorant work for their own profit, Arjuna; the wise work for the welfare of the world, without thought for themselves.[1]

Having a grounded spiritual practice to support us can completely shift our relationship to the world. It can change the way we take care of our own body, the way we speak to our children, the way we vote, how engaged we are with our community—if we are strong enough to speak up for those that are suffering—and generally, how we serve in the world. Our practice is a microcosm for the way we exist in the world. It's a field for us to resolve inner confusion so that we can see clearly and engage in the world in a more conscious way.

You don't have to be an activist, or social justice warrior, to engage in the teachings this way. In fact, this is not a question of altruism or doing good deeds. It's about your own spiritual awakening and reducing your own suffering. The point is that if you think of other people, and the way your actions affect them, you are the one who benefits in the end. Your own service, kindness, and compassion will create a happier and more joyful life for yourself. Of course, it also creates a more harmonious world for all of us.

## COMMUNITY CARE

We can learn so much from nature about how to care for ourselves and for others. Recent research indicates that trees have vast underground "wood wide webs" of fungal (mycorrhizal) networks.

> By analyzing the DNA in root tips and tracing the movement of molecules through underground conduits, [the researcher Suzanne] Simard has discovered that fungal threads link nearly every tree in a forest—even trees of different species. Carbon, water, nutrients, alarm signals and hormones can pass from tree to tree through these subterranean circuits. Resources tend to flow from the oldest and biggest trees to the youngest and smallest. Chemical alarm signals generated by one tree prepare nearby trees for danger. Seedlings severed from the forest's underground lifelines are much more likely to die than their networked counterparts. And if a tree is on the brink of death, it sometimes bequeaths a substantial share of its carbon to its neighbors.[2]

For the last few years the term "community care" has been used by social justice activists, and through the COVID-19 pandemic we got to see it put into practice. We also got to see the obstacles to community care. Mask wearing and social distancing are forms of community care because those actions put the benefit of others over your own. By staying home and wearing masks we were taking care of people with compromised immune systems and seniors, two groups that were the most susceptible to the virus. Community care also means creating mutual support networks. These networks are generally organized by neighborhood and include checking in on elderly neighbors and setting up networks for sharing resources and information.

Like "mother trees" in vast forest networks that generously share their resources, we were caring for those who didn't have access to health care or the privilege of going a few weeks without pay when they got sick. Times of crisis offer an opportunity to explore the connection between the individual and the community.

> Who is in your community? Do you have a local network of friends and neighbors? Do you have a digital community? How do you contribute to this community? Can you make this contribution part of your yoga practice?

## APART BUT TOGETHER

Sitting in silence together in group meditation has taught me more about community than all the parties and dinners I've ever attended. I've literally sat in hundreds, if not thousands, of group meditations as well as meditations at the end of countless yoga classes. The power of the group stills my mind and opens my heart. When I sit in meditation alone, I crave the container of the group to hold me. Sometimes I imagine that I'm surrounded by other meditators so I can feel their presence and, with their support, go deep within.

In silence, I open myself to the truth of our shared essence—love. It sounds like a cliché, but it all comes down to love. And that is what is so confusing. Love is what we call the romantic feelings we have for our partner, and it's the same word we use for the most intimate connected spirit, or self meeting itself.

When I get quiet, just for a moment, I can feel your heart. It's just like mine, although you are completely different than I am. Your life, your struggles, your pain and happiness may be unknown to me, but I know your heart. Like light through a prism, our consciousness is the same, but our manifestation is different. We're all the colors of the rainbow, and yet we're simply pure white light.

> Consider the relationship between your body-mind and your spirit. When you act, do you consider who is acting? When you move, who is moving? Can you integrate spirit into the reality of the seen world? Try to do one action as if your spirit is doing it instead of your body and mind. It could be walking across the room or reaching for a glass of water and taking a sip. Feel like your spirit is moving through you, and your body is the vehicle.

## RECONCILING SELF-CARE AND SERVICE

The tension between self-care and community care is one of the biggest challenges facing contemporary yoga. The fact that we have to be told to care for others is an interesting dilemma, not only within yoga communities, but in society in general. An example of this dilemma is the argument over wearing masks during COVID, or using condoms to fight AIDS, both of which speak to the idea of self-sacrifice for the benefit of others. It reminds me of that quote that was falsely attributed to Anthony Fauci, but was actually by the writer Lauren Morrill, "I don't know how to explain to you why you should care about other people."[3]

This tension is found in the fact that the teachings generally focus on the goal of samadhi, enlightenment, without understanding the relationship between the individual and the community. The practice of service, karma yoga or seva, is one of the paths of yoga described in the Gita that seems almost completely lost today. In our contemporary society there is such a strong emphasis on the individual—often at the expense of the community—that these teachings have been lost or twisted to support a system that relies on competition and productivity over all else.

The concept of wellness, in particular, has been used by the capitalist system to distort a spiritual practice in the service of profit. Often, workers are taught that through wellness and self-care they will become more effective and more productive. This is taking a community problem—namely, not taking care of each other with proper health care, sick leave, parental leave, and so on—and putting the burden back on individuals to take care of themselves. It's an interesting paradox, because the practices of yoga do offer individual empowerment. But the practices of self-care don't replace the need for the community to care for those who are struggling.

According to the anonymous rebel alliance, CrimethInc: "Wherever a value is considered universal, we find the pressures of normativity: for example, the pressure to perform self-care for others' sake, keeping up appearances. So much of what we do in this society is about maintaining the image that we're successful, autonomous individuals, regardless of the reality. In this context, rhetoric about self-care can mask silencing and policing: Deal with your problems yourself, please, so no one else has to."[4]

## PERFORMANCE AND ABLEISM

Yoga is often used by contemporary capitalist culture to perpetuate the status quo. We are expected to perform in yoga classes, which are often competitive environments that value perfectionism and conformity over individual agency and healing. We have to ask ourselves who is being served by this competitive, performative yoga space? Is it the student or the business that benefits from this model? Unfortunately, contemporary yoga's popularity is largely based on competition to see who can look successful and happy. But these goals are antithetical to the spiritual teachings of yoga, which value nonattachment and service above all else.

> Ask yourself, is the goal of your yoga practice your personal liberation or the liberation of others? If your practice is about your own healing, is there a way to expand your thinking to include healing for your community, your society, and the entire planet? What would that look like in practice?

I recently read an account from a yoga student who shared about the painful experiences she had in yoga in a Facebook post. She explained, "My yoga teachers shamed me for my appearance. I wasn't so lucky when it comes to the physical body, and I've been struggling with that. It took me years just to do asanas again, and even today I can't talk about it."

I found this comment devastating for so many reasons, not the least of which is because it's a common experience that I've heard too many times. Not only had her teachers failed to practice yoga themselves, but they were acting in an unethical manner. Shaming someone and making them feel that they're not, "lucky when it comes to the physical body," is antithetical to the teachings. Yoga is not about physical achievement, rather it's about identifying with spirit. I say it repeatedly, and hopefully someone is listening: advanced yoga is not advanced yoga asana!

In fact, the way we have equated advanced practice with physical ability is a form of deeply ingrained ableism. Ableism is the incorrect notion that some bodies are better than other bodies, as well as the idea that disabled bodies need to be fixed or healed. We are trained from a young age that disability, illness, old age, fatness, and any other differences from some supposed norm are to be avoided and shamed.

I often wonder what wellness looks like without ableism? For that matter, what would yoga practice look like without the influence of ableism? Can we even imagine a contemporary practice where we remove those corrupted ideas and where asana isn't the goal? In many ways, that's what I'm trying to find in this book. I'm searching for a yoga that is truly universal, rather than a yoga that perpetuates white supremacist and capitalist notions of health, achievement, and wellness. For me, an advanced yoga practitioner isn't someone who can stand on their head, but someone who is at peace with themselves and offering service in the world.

As De Jur Jones shares, she is offering yoga to incarcerated and formerly incarcerated people who don't see themselves in yoga. They come to her class because all bodies are welcome. By creating a welcoming space, her students experience tremendous benefit from the practice, including feeling, "a bit better," and walking out with yoga tools.

## PAINFUL OR PAINLESS THOUGHTS

There is an important concept that relates to this focus beyond the individual in the beginning of the Yoga Sutras, just after we're introduced to the basic theme of working to still the mind and connect with spirit. In chapter 1, sutra 5, Patanjali describes all the different kinds of thoughts that exist in our mind. It's a powerful statement; he explains that all our thoughts can be divided into just five types.

He goes on to say that those five types of thought can actually be broken down further into just two main categories. All thought can be categorized in two ways—either causing suffering, *klishta*, or not causing suffering, *aklishta*. So, in order to work with the thoughts, we first need to analyze them and understand what they are made of.

This is a powerful teaching that is echoed later in the second chapter, when Patanjali offers one of the most relieving statements in all of yoga: "Future suffering is avoidable." It's also echoed in the Gita, when Krishna explains that the path of yoga is about stopping our identification with that which experiences suffering. The real questions are: "What is it that causes this suffering?" and, "How can we avoid it?" It's so interesting to reflect on

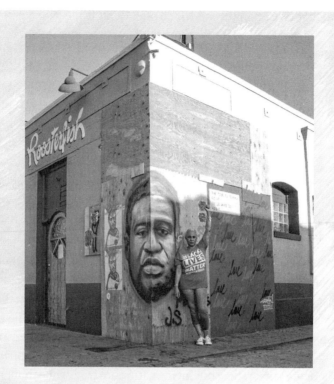

## DE JUR JONES

I chose to be of service as a volunteer yoga teacher to bring yoga therapy to incarcerated and formerly incarcerated people around Los Angeles County, California. These forgotten communities really thrived from their Accessible Yoga programs. For many of them, prison or jail was the gateway to first hearing of or practicing yoga. Many of them go on to have a home practice and seek out community classes upon release once they get on their feet. In my classes, all bodies are welcome. I ask people to bring their cellmates and friends, even those that did not feel like "doing" yoga. They were invited to rest during the entire class. It brought me such joy when students shared that something that was physically bothering them when they entered class felt a bit better, and they walked out with yoga tools to treat this issue in the future.

which thoughts are painful and which ones don't bring pain. Personally, I know which ones I want! But how much of our practice is spent reflecting on this essential question?

Take a moment to reflect on your thoughts, and see if you can notice their impact. Which thoughts are painful? Which ones don't bring pain?

The answer is a little more complicated than it may seem on the surface. It's not simply that big emotions like anger or selfishness cause pain. We have to go back to Patanjali's fundamental philosophy, rather than use our contemporary mindset to understand. He says that when the thoughts are stilled, we will experience the fullness of the true self, spirit, atman, or purusha, whichever word you prefer. So, we need to understand thought as something that can either disturb the mind or not disturb the mind, as something that blocks our view or something that allows the mind to see the truth.

In many ways, yoga is a practice of truthfulness, satya. The truth is we are spiritual beings having this temporary human experience. Truthful thoughts reflect the universal love that is the nature of our spiritual essence. Thoughts that reflect our loving nature are true, while thoughts that are based on attachments, or external, limited things, aren't true. Truthful thoughts don't cause pain, while thoughts that are based on lies cause pain. The lies of yoga are the many ways we look outside of our own heart for happiness or fulfillment. Pain comes when we are externally focused, looking for validation or love to come from outside of us. Painless, truthful thoughts are those that reflect our spiritual nature, compassionate thoughts like: "I care about you," "I love you," "Are you okay?" "How can I support you?"

Cultivating these painless thoughts, based in the truth of our spirit, is the foundation of karma yoga. We get to align our actions in the world with the truth of our heart. We can act out of love and compassion for others. Of course, it's not as easy as it sounds. We may not have trouble acting in a loving way toward our family or dear friends. But can we expand our hearts to bring that loving, truthful vision to the way we see the rest of the world?

According to the writer Rachel Naomi Remen, "Fixing and helping create a distance between people, but we cannot serve at a distance. We can only serve that to which we are profoundly connected."[5] The gift of service is connection, not allowing ourselves to be above or below anyone else. It is not fixing or helping, but being present, equal, and awake.

## YOGA IN ACTION

Service provides a way to bring yoga into all my daily activities by asking me to be constantly alert to my mind and the ways that my ego inserts itself into most situations. I don't want to overly criticize the ego-mind, because it's an essential part of myself, but I do want to find a way to practice yoga internally that allows me to stretch and strengthen my mind. A strong mind and healthy ego will allow me to be more effective in the world and truly be of service—by not making everything about me!

There are many ways that I see yoga expanding our hearts and helping us live a life of service. One way is that yoga offers us tools for personal exploration and self-study. This helps us in understanding our own position and privilege. It's the heart of Patanjali's teaching of kriya yoga, yoga in action, which I discussed briefly before, but I think is worth reviewing since it's the key to karma yoga. It's interesting to note that both *karma* and *kriya* derive from the Sanskrit word for "to do." Remember, kriya yoga has three steps: tapas, learning from suffering; svadhyaya, reflection; and ishvarapranidhana, surrender.

I see tapas as the openness to learn from challenges and suffering. It's the reaction to pain that goes something like, "Oh no! Here I go again. I got upset by that same thing." It's the willingness to consider that the suffering of life can teach us something, rather than simply responding in kind with something like, "No, it's not me, it's you!"

Svadhyaya is reflection, or self-study. It's the willingness to look at *why* we got upset, and the acknowledgment that our own attachments are at the root of all our suffering. In other words, it's admitting that our continued effort to find happiness and fulfillment in the external world has caused us to suffer. Of course, external circumstances can lead to suffering as well, so we need to be careful here. But it's the realization that our own patterns can lead us to repeat the same mistakes over and over again, until we're willing to learn a lesson.

This reminds me of my current struggles trying to parent teenagers. As much as I'm attached to their happiness, they are continually reminding me that it's none of my business. When they act out, or get upset with me, it's usually because they're telling me, "I'm not your baby anymore. Treat me like an adult. Don't use me to fulfill whatever needs you have." Svadhyaya means I'm willing to hear this message and reflect on my role as a parent. Am I attached to that role, or am I willing to allow my role to change and grow as my children do?

The last step of kriya yoga, yoga in action, is ishvarapranidhana, surrender to God, or spirit. Remember, in the yoga tradition, God is not an external person, but rather accessible within us. This isn't about surrendering to an old man sitting on a cloud. Rather, it's surrendering to our inner essence. Surrender is being true to ourselves. It's also about finally admitting that the peace, joy, and fulfillment that I'm searching for are actually already within me, as me.

Together, the three aspects of kriya yoga work in a special choreography of spiritual growth and learning; three steps to gaining inner wisdom and greater awareness. This is how we take yoga off the mat and apply the teachings in our lives. It works like this:

1. Tapas: If you get upset about something—maybe someone criticizes you, and you feel hurt—you pause and think, "Time for yoga!"
2. Svadhyaya: Can you ask yourself, "Why did I get upset by that? What am I attached to in this situation?"
3. Ishvarapranidhana: Consider, "Can I let it go? Do I trust that I'm okay, and that the sacred peace within me is untouched by this situation?"

Karma yoga is walking a conscious spiritual path in the world, and kriya yoga offers signposts along that path. Personally, service is the form my yoga practice has taken. But, it's an extremely challenging path in so many ways, so I'm hesitant to even say it out loud! Not only is it challenging to stay true to the spiritual vision that yoga demands of me, it's also challenging to not fall into the sticky traps of my ego-mind and become stranded in my attachments.

Attachments, as I mentioned earlier, are the obstacles to the truth. They are what we see when we practice svadhyaya: the lies we tell ourselves all the time, the lies that actually interfere with our spiritual awakening and build up the ego's false sense of self. But who doesn't want to get compliments, approval, acknowledgment, and more Instagram likes? It's human nature, often based in our survival instincts, that leads us to seek external validation, and that's why spiritual life is so challenging. Perhaps the most important question of yoga is, "Can I find value in myself, rather than in the opinions of others?"

> How much do I depend on validation from others for my own peace of mind? Are there particular areas in my life where I am more dependent than others?

## HOW TO SERVE

Karma yoga means acting without attachment to the result of our actions, without thinking about how our actions will fulfill our selfish desires. What's confusing about this is the role of survival and self-care. Are those selfish desires? We have to care for ourselves before we can offer service in the world. How do we find the line between survival, self-care, and service?

I think the answer is that self-care is service to the body and mind. Self-care is not about spoiling ourselves occasionally; it's about making conscious choices to protect our energy, our health, and our peace of mind. Boundaries are the best form of self-care. They allow us to focus on what the body and mind need to flourish, rather than what other people think we need or what other people need from us.

Yoga practice helps us to see this more clearly. The practices are designed to give us an unbreakable bond with the most intimate part of ourselves. Through practice, we can see through the untruths that we have told ourselves and, with kindness, change our thinking to reflect the truth of who we are. Karma yoga means we are open to learning from our actions in the world. We start to see where we have attachments and expectations from even the smallest interactions: "Why did he cut me off?" "Why didn't she say thank you?" "Doesn't he appreciate me?"

Having a regular yoga practice can help us build resilience—physically, emotionally, and mentally. So when challenges come, we can take that momentary pause and practice kriya yoga. It can take time, and we don't have to be perfect at it. Even recognizing an attachment just one time will bring tremendous benefit.

I think of my formal practices of meditation, pranayama, and asana as preparation for the service I do in the world. Those formal practices are the way I care for myself so I can serve more effectively, and they help me get into the right frame of mind to serve. I always try to remember that service isn't about what I'm doing as much as the way I'm doing it.

This is the conundrum of spiritual practice: Can I work on myself and contribute to the greater good? The answer is yes, if I practice karma yoga. I do this by looking at my life and seeing where there is tension or a need and putting my energy there without getting caught up in needing a specific result. We don't have to travel to another country to serve people in need. We can look at our closest relationships—our friends, coworkers, neighbors, and students—to find an outlet for our service.

## SPIRITUAL POWER WITHOUT SERVICE IS SIMPLY POWER

Service in the world can take the form of social justice, even though many people aren't comfortable with that terminology. So, I'll just say that for me, personally, social justice is where I see my work in the world and where I get to practice service. But social justice may not be everyone's path. Each of us has our own battles to fight and our own purpose, or dharma, to fulfill.

I think this is the missing piece of contemporary yoga practice. Right now, it seems like most yoga practitioners are using their practice to feel better, get healthier, and build energy. They're focusing on their own wellness. The question is, what do you do with all that energy? If you don't work on the mind, then that extra energy from your practice may just amplify what's already going on inside of you.

Remember, spiritual power without service is simply power. Service is an outlet for your energy. It allows the energy that you build in your practice to be used for the greater good—not just for your own personal benefit. This focus on others, and not simply expanding your own ego, is really at the basis of spiritual practice. So, it's not a matter of right or wrong, but a question of effective vs. ineffective spiritual practice. It's a paradox: the more I serve you, the happier I will be.

We even see this in animals. A recent study of rats showed that they naturally cared for each other. They would avoid actions that hurt other rats, even if it would offer them a reward.[6] Again, service to ourselves has to come first. I can imagine that the rats were also taking care that they weren't being hurt themselves. We need to fulfill our own needs before we offer service in the world, and it's a lifelong challenge to find the balance between self-care and service.

I see so many examples of service in the world around me every day. I look at people in the service professions who are committed to their work. I remember when, years ago, I was in the hospital for some minor surgery, and I was blown away by the way that the nurses and staff were there for me when I couldn't care for myself. I could feel that they authentically cared for me. It changed my experience of being so vulnerable and allowed me to relax. They were acting with love and compassion, which is the heart of service.

Service can also be practiced outside of obvious service jobs. I used to be a professional gardener, and I remember how gardening became a practice for me. I would try to focus on how the plants could benefit—were they in the correct location, were they getting the right amount of water, the right kind of soil? Some days I felt present with the plants in a way that's hard to describe. I think that is the gift of service: present-moment awareness and peace of mind. Of course, some days it was horrible. I was working outside in the rain and mud, my back would hurt, and I didn't have anywhere I could pee. It's not all or nothing. Those moments of bliss were few and far between, but I cherished them.

Most yoga teachers are practicing service when they teach, whether it's to special populations or a studio class. Most of us know that teaching yoga isn't really a very profitable profession, but we do it for the love of yoga and the love of our students. Teaching yoga is a great way to love other people, and service is love in action. This can be true whether we're getting paid to teach or volunteering. You can get paid for a job and it can be service if you have the right attitude. In fact, you can volunteer and it isn't service if you expect that "thank you" afterwards. The ego's needs are tricky and it can find its way into almost any situation. That's why karma yoga is an entire path of yoga and a lifelong practice.

In my experience, the service state of mind is transitory but profound. It's a feeling of openness and connection with others. Actually, we have the

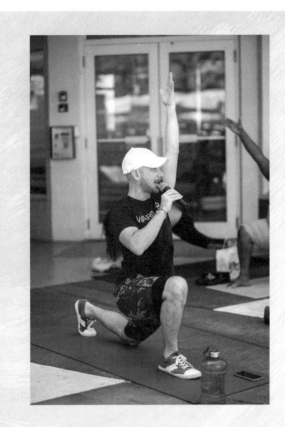

**ADRIAN MOLINA**

After teaching commercial yoga for many years, my heart pulled me in a different direction. I went through some difficult chapters in my personal life, but the practice stood next to me, reflecting back. I learned different ways to relate to the practice of yoga, and different ways to share the teachings. I longed to share the practice in unconventional places, with underserved audiences: homeless shelters, hospitals, police and fire stations, and more. I wanted the practice to bring hope to those who felt forgotten, because I had been there once. I never thought the practice of yoga would become my doorway into social justice. But these days, I can't see one without the other.

opportunity to practice service in every waking moment. As I said, it's a state of mind more than a specific activity. Service is acting without a selfish motivation. If you have limited energy or means, you can offer service by mentally offering the benefit of your actions for others or the world around you. This is dedication in action. Can you think kindly of someone or send them some positive energy? Even in the context of your daily action you can practice this kind of dedicated service. Can you walk across the room in a way that respects your body, your shoes, the floorboards, and the space above and below you? Being present in your body as you move in the world is an important service.

In order to be of service you need to start with self-awareness. Notice your thoughts as you are doing a simple action. As I sweep the floor, am I aware of the way I am sweeping or caught up in my mind? If I can focus on the work in front of me with all my attention, that is service.

My favorite form of service is listening. When someone talks to me I try to notice my mind's tendency to start coming up with answers before they're done or to think of how what they're saying affects me. I practice service by listening to what they're saying and giving them my full attention. It is also a beautiful practice to try to put yourself in someone else's shoes. Next time you're having a disagreement with someone try to pause and think about how they feel and why. Working with the mind in this way is a subtle and powerful way to practice service.

> Engage in active listening. The next time you're listening to someone see if you can watch the way your mind reacts. Can you fully listen to what they're saying before thinking of a response?

# 9 | PRACTICE IN REAL LIFE

AT A FAMOUS PRESS conference in 1982, when over 1,000 Americans had already died of AIDS, then president Reagan's press secretary, Larry Speakes, made homophobic jokes with reporters about the epidemic, which he called the "gay plague."[1] It was a time that felt oddly similar to the coronavirus pandemic. The difference was that AIDS is a sexually transmitted disease that was mostly affecting gay men. It was originally named GRID (gay-related immunodeficiency disease). You can imagine society's reaction to that.

There was a lot of fear, victim blaming, and harassment of people with HIV and AIDS. Homophobia definitely fed into the lack of response and general apathy to the epidemic from the public as well as from the government. Ronald Reagan refused to even mention the word *AIDS* publicly for four years after the first cases appeared. He literally wouldn't even talk about it.

This type of inhumane callousness was unbearable for me. I was distraught about my friends getting sick and dying, so I dedicated myself to speaking out and drawing attention to the devastation that was happening in my community. I ended up organizing and marching in countless protests and getting arrested multiple times. I didn't feel like I had a voice or any way to bring awareness to what was happening, so it was the least I could do.

It's interesting to consider how my activism was a form of service. Blocking traffic, painting signs, marching in the streets, and getting arrested were all ways for me to express my love for my community. From the outside, I can see how these kinds of angry protests might not look like love in action, but that's what they are. We took ACT UP's slogan, Silence = Death, to heart and screamed for our survival—for someone to pay attention and show some human decency. It took years before the government had a decent response to AIDS, and by that time it was too late. The virus had spread all over the world and killed hundreds of thousands of gay men, as well as many other people from marginalized communities. Even today,

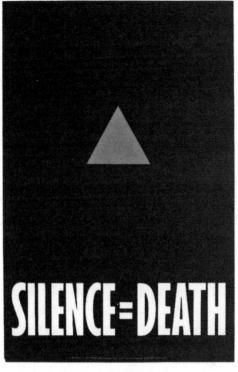

Silence = Death Poster[2]

there is no vaccine or cure for AIDS, and thousands of people continue to be infected every day.[3]

## HAVING CHILDREN

I met my husband, Matt, through ACT UP, and luckily he shared my passion for activism. After Matt and I had been together for a number of years, we decided to pursue having children. We felt that our existence as a queer family would be a form of protest in itself, showing the world that we survived when so many of our friends didn't. To survive, and thrive, as a marginalized person is a powerful statement.

This was around the year 2000. At the time, we didn't think gay adoption was legal, since gay marriage was still not legal in the United States. We heard that open adoption was one way we could create a family. It was also a relatively new concept, but it seemed like a perfect option for us because it's based on the idea of honesty and choice. The main idea is that the birthparents choose the adoptive parents for their child, and then ongoing contact is negotiated directly between them.

We loved the simple logic of birthparents deciding on the placement of their child, and decided to pursue it. We completed an exhaustive home study, and were told it would take about two years. But, within two weeks we met our son's birthmother, who at the time was five months pregnant. We were so excited to get to spend time with her, and she became part of our extended family.

Since I was a yoga teacher and a gardener, and made very little money, Matt and I decided that I should be the stay-at-home parent, and he would continue with his nine-to-five job so that we could live off of his salary. In the end, I had the incredible opportunity of raising both our children from birth—an experience that few men get to have.

All I can say is, "Phew!" Parenting is service. It is love in action. Waking up in the middle of the night multiple times to feed and change an infant is a mind-bending experience. The constant care needed for infants, and children in general, takes a huge heart and very caring mind. We eventually adopted our daughter through open adoption as well, and now they're both teenagers, which is another story altogether!

As I've heard other people describe it, parenting is like walking around with your heart outside of your body. I didn't realize how self-absorbed I was until I had to think of my kids so much. I'm not complaining, because children are an amazing gift, but the challenge is real. Parenting my kids was especially intense because of my daughter's mental health challenges. So I should add that parenting a kid with disabilities is a special challenge that really pushed me to my limits. It's an invisible struggle that can often feel isolating and hopeless. To other parents of kids with disabilities, I just want to say that I see you.

## THE LOCKS AND KEYS OF PARENTING

After a few years of parenting, I started to realize that the yoga teachings were a powerful tool not just for my self-care, but for helping me parent. So often I found that my yoga practice offered me space in my mind to consider how to respond to a situation. Meditation, pranayama, and asana all helped me become less reactive. But sometimes that backfired. I remember thinking, "I shouldn't let my kids talk to me like that," instead of simply responding with a "no way!"

One of the tools I found most effective was a single sutra from the Yoga Sutras (1.33), which my teacher called the Locks and Keys. This sutra says:

> By cultivating attitudes of friendliness toward the happy, com-passion for the unhappy, delight in the virtuous, and equanimity toward the non-virtuous, the mind-stuff retains its undisturbed calmness.[4]

The name "Locks and Keys" refers to the idea that there are four kinds of situations we often face in the world (or sometimes in our own mind)—these are the locks. The sutra says there is a correct way to respond to those situations and these are the keys to those locks. In a way, it's misleading to say these are the "correct" responses. The point of the yoga teachings isn't simply doing the correct action so much as considering what makes an action correct. These "keys" allow us to "unlock," or navigate, challenging situations with ease.

The last part of this sutra is worth noting. It explains that by using these keys, "the mind-stuff retains its undisturbed calmness." This is a powerful teaching about the nature of the mind. Often, I feel like my mind is com-pletely out of control—whether spinning, obsessing, or planning. This statement about the mind returning to an undisturbed calm is such a relief.

I love the idea that my mind is calm by nature, and that it has some-how been disturbed. It reminds me of sediment in vinegar. If you mix it up it becomes cloudy, and you can't see through it. If you let it settle, the sediment falls to the bottom and the liquid becomes clear. What a relief that Patanjali thinks our minds are, by nature, calm. That alone affected my ability to parent: I could use my practice to continue to return to that place within me, undisturbed by the chaos in the world of kids. Of course, just finding time for practice was a challenge.

Over the past few years since my mother passed away, I've been focus-ing on mothering myself. These tools have become a lifeline for me and have helped me take care of myself. In fact, I would suggest that the Locks and

Keys may be the essence of self-care. They are showing us how to create boundaries when we're facing challenging situations and difficult people. Most of our stress and anxiety is related to dealing with other people, so this is no small feat.

Boundaries are an interesting and essential theme in the yoga teachings, and they're rarely discussed in this context. Yoga is about finding that fine line between compassion and codependency. We learn how to take care of ourselves, and by doing so we become less reliant on others. We expand our hearts and also our ability to see when we're being abused, neglected, or overly dependent on others. Yoga is self-care, and as I noted before, self-care is service to ourselves. We take care of ourselves first, and then we can care for others. That's a hard lesson I learned from parenting—and one I continue to learn.

Can you think of a time when you didn't have boundaries and you thought you were being loving and compassionate? Reflect on the balance between being openhearted and allowing yourself to be in an abusive situation.

## FRIENDLINESS TOWARD THE HAPPY

I found the Locks and Keys very effective tools for parenting, and I needed all the help I could get. They offered guidance for working with the minds of my children and responding to them in a way that would support them while allowing my mind to "retain its undisturbed calmness."

The first lock is "friendliness toward the happy." I think the point here is the benefit of having a relatively neutral response toward another person's happiness. It means we don't rely on other people's happiness for our happiness, which I found to be a huge hurdle as a parent. I was very attached to my kids' happiness, and to be honest, I still am! It's a lesson in boundaries.

When my kids were little, I began to see how sensitive I was to their emotions, and that I needed to keep some perspective. I needed the neutrality of "friendliness" to their emotions rather than joining them in their feelings. Part of that was simply trying to keep my head above water in what often seemed like a sea of chaos, but it was also a lesson in human relationships. We don't really know why someone is happy. It could be that they just tripped their sibling or because they cheated them in a game. Also, we don't want to be happy just because someone else is happy, instead we can try to remember the truth of yoga: our happiness arises from inside of us. Otherwise, we're being codependent.

> Can you think of a situation where friendliness toward the happy would help you keep your peace?

## COMPASSION FOR THE UNHAPPY

"Compassion for the unhappy" is an incredibly powerful concept, providing a path to our own peace of mind through caring for others. Compassion helps us to retain our undisturbed calmness. Here's a statement I'd like to plaster on walls and yell from mountaintops: "Compassion *brings* peace." It is in loving and serving others, in seeing ourselves in others, that we fulfill ourselves. In many ways this statement reflects the underlying theme of this book: yoga practice as social justice.

This was usually an easy one for me. I could soothe my children when they were sad or hurt. I had compassion when they expressed their unhappiness to me, but I had to be careful here too. It was easy to go too far. Sometimes expressing unhappiness is simply whining or complaining, or sometimes it's an honest expression of pain that doesn't need a response. I learned to clarify my responses, "I am sorry you're feeling sad, or upset, but that doesn't mean you'll get whatever it is you're whining for." This was a boundary I was always looking for.

I saw that it was possible to lose myself in my compassion for my kids. I remember my son coming home from school and complaining about the way some other child had treated him. My first response was to jump to his defense. But, after asking more details about the interaction I saw that my son hadn't been very nice either. Generally, I learned that I could have compassion for however they were feeling without necessarily basing my actions on their emotions.

The same is true for myself. If I'm feeling upset or sad about something, I try to respect my emotions and the powerful energy they bring, without necessarily acting on them. In other words, thank God for email drafts! It's one thing to write someone an angry response when they've hurt your feelings, but it's another thing to send it. Compassion for myself means that I give my emotions lots of respect without allowing them to control important decisions in my life. I have an agreement with myself that I won't make decisions when I'm upset. Instead, I'll wait until the emotion has passed, and then make a decision. This has saved me from a lot of bad decisions in my life.

> Making hard decisions: When faced with making a difficult decision, see if it's possible to pull out the emotion from the facts of the situation. Seeing the emotion as valuable is important, because that's the language of your heart. But that doesn't have to be the end of the story.

There's a beautiful passage in the Gita that speaks to this idea of emotion clouding judgment. Arjuna is questioning Krishna about what it means to be a steady person—a yogi. Krishna describes the way that we are tossed about by conflicting emotions and opinions all the time. He describes the path that we take to losing our discerning mind and how to find true peace.

> When a man dwells on the pleasures of sense, attraction for them arises in him. From attraction arises desire, the lust of possession, and this leads to passion, to anger.
>
> From passion comes confusion of mind, then loss of remembrance, the forgetting of duty. From this loss comes the ruin of reason, and the ruin of reason leads man to destruction.
>
> But the soul that moves in the world of the senses and yet keeps the senses in harmony, free from attraction and aversion, finds rest in quietness.
>
> In this quietness falls down the burden of all her sorrows, for when the heart has found quietness, wisdom has also found peace.
>
> There is no wisdom for a man without harmony, and without harmony there is no contemplation. Without contemplation there cannot be peace, and without peace can there be joy?[5]

There is something about that passage that almost brings me to tears every time I read it, and I'm not sure why. I think it's because it describes so powerfully the ways that we get lost. This translation by Juan Mascaro is particularly powerful, and there are so many jewels here. I love the section,

"In this quietness falls down the burden of all her sorrows, for when the heart has found quietness, wisdom has also found peace." It's interesting how well this message from the Gita connects to the main teaching of the Yoga Sutras regarding quieting the mind and allowing the heart to be free.

This is one of the secret powers that yoga offers—the ability to be resilient enough to feel our strongest feelings. According to Michelle Cassandra Johnson, this is also the way to make social change—through feeling, not through thinking:

> If we are going to make social change, we need to cultivate a practice of feeling. If someone could think us out of the social injustice that we are swimming in, a very smart someone would have done so by now. When one connects with their feelings as yoga teaches us to do, they can connect with their heart. If one is connected with their heart, they have the opportunity to be changed and to shift their perspective. They have the opportunity to feel the pain of living in a world that is designed to break the spirit through violence, oppression and injustice. Feeling the pain, individually and, more importantly, collectively allows for us to grieve, to acknowledge and truth tell and to aspire to be better than the legacy that white supremacy has left us.[6]

Can I offer myself compassion when I am suffering? What would that look like in my life?

## DELIGHT IN THE VIRTUOUS

This lock and key may be the most directly related to parenting. I can think of so many times I reached for this tool. In many ways, this idea of "delighting in the virtuous" is simply a matter of focusing energy on the thing that you want to grow or expand. It's about giving children positive affirmations when they act in a loving or generous way. I remember all those times my kids would do something beautiful. They would save a small bug by carefully carrying it outside, or care for me when I was hurt, or question why people would act in a mean way. Children are born with loving hearts, and so often, the world hardens them.

Delighting in the virtuous is also a profound teaching for spiritual practitioners, as well as social justice warriors. It's easy to get discouraged when
we're fighting for truth and equity, and to feel that evil is winning. By delighting in the virtuous we can focus our minds on the positive steps that
are happening. This isn't about being in denial—we'll get to that next—but
about focusing on the positive, on those small positive improvements that
inspire us to keep fighting and keep moving forward.

In our spiritual practice, this can mean focusing on the inspirational,
generous, loving people that we see around us every day. That way, if we
focus on them enough, we'll begin to emulate their behavior. We are such
social creatures and so highly influenced by those around us. Even on social
media, I see the positive influence we can have on each other. Every day,
I see people cheering each other on, congratulating each other for their
successes, and generally being supportive and concerned. That inspires
me to be more supportive and virtuous myself. This is one of the reasons
why community is so essential for spiritual growth. By surrounding yourself with people who share your ethics and priorities, you'll continually be
inspired by them to stay focused.

## EQUANIMITY TOWARD THE NON-VIRTUOUS

Social media offers many opportunities to practice this last lock and key,
"equanimity toward the non-virtuous." It's really a matter of trying to keep
my sanity in the Wild West of social media. I've had to unfollow, and even
block, people who post offensive or mean things. I find that blocking or
deleting is a better response than engaging in a fight. This feels like a way
to practice equanimity toward non-virtuous behavior. The times when I
have argued with people online have never ended well. These arguments
tend to spiral out of control, and usually don't offer any productive results,
other than a lot of stress.

It's not that I don't speak my mind on social media, I sure do! But I don't
do it in opposition to others. I do it in a way that can educate and uplift people
to find a more compassionate view of the world. In this way, I keep my peace
of mind and help further the conversation. In-person interactions are different than online ones, so this is really my commentary on how to navigate
the world of social media in a way that spreads a positive message and allows

me to keep my peace. And that is the point of this last key—equanimity. If I can stay neutral and not react, I can be more effective in creating change.

Arguing with angry people often feels like yelling fire in a crowded theater: it just creates more panic rather than leading to any kind of growth or resolution. On the other hand, this teaching could be used to excuse spiritual bypassing, which I'll discuss in detail later. But that's not the point of equanimity toward non-virtuous behavior. It's not asking us to ignore our own painful emotions or the pain of others. (Remember, the key to understanding our own suffering or the suffering of others is to have compassion.)

Instead, this teaching is asking us to walk away from confrontation. It reminds me of a quote from Michelle Obama, "When I hear about negative and false attacks, I really don't invest any energy in them, because I know who I am."[7] Finding equanimity when under attack allows us to stay true to our essence, which is peace. The power of her statement, "I know who I am," really rings in my heart. Once I know who I am other people don't affect me in the same way. I'm not looking for other people to fill me up.

My kids helped me understand the true meaning of this teaching when they were little. When they did something mean or selfish, it was easy to put a lot of attention on what they were doing wrong. Instead, I tried to keep my equanimity in response to unkind or mean behavior. I found that it was more effective to redirect their energy to something more productive, and that would help to extinguish the behavior.

I remember one time I picked up my daughter from preschool and she was covered from head to toe in finger paint. I could see that she was nervous and expected me to be upset with her. I think she was testing me. Instead, I basically said, "If you had used paper we could have hung your paintings on the wall. Now it's all going to go down the drain in the bathtub."

Keeping my head on straight when things were out of control was my main job when my kids were little. I was always running after someone or refereeing some argument between them. I remember one time my kids were yelling at each other, and I just started yelling nonsense really loudly. Soon we all ended up laughing about it. The beauty of this teaching is that it helps us see our own judgmental nature. If we keep our peace during conflict we can keep everyone safe, and help to bring the cool rain of peace when every last drop of calm has evaporated.

## 10 | THE EVOLUTION OF OUR PRACTICE

IT'S FUN TO EXPLORE yoga poses, to get the body moving and begin to notice the movement of breath and energy. But it's important to remember that yoga is so much more than poses. It's not just the perfect alignment of Triangle Pose, Trikonasana, and obsessing over whether the hip should be forward or back. Instead, it's aligning the heart and head. Specifically, yoga is transcending the mind's power trip that keeps us lost and confused. Often I don't know which voice in my head is ego and which is spirit. My mind feels more like spin art, a mess of colors, images, and worries. But I do know what it feels like to *not* be in my head—that active stillness that comes during Shavasana or occasionally in meditation. It's that lightness I feel after I practice.

Why does yoga make me feel so much better? Maybe it's because it gives me temporary relief from the constant whirling in my head? Maybe it's a pause on that trip my ego is on? But what is this ego that we're always talking about in yoga? Meditation teacher Sally Kempton beautifully describes the ups and downs of the ego to a ride on a seesaw:

> It is this tendency to identify with our thoughts and feelings about ourselves and the world that creates the problem of ego. If we could let thoughts and feelings pass through us, we wouldn't get insulted, or nurse hurt feelings, or worry about whether we were smart enough or worthy enough. In short, we wouldn't spend our time riding the emotional seesaw that's the backdrop of most people's days.
>
> Recently I spent several days monitoring this pattern, and I was fascinated to see how much of my inner life is a ride on that seesaw. I'd wake up after an expansive dream and feel good about myself. I'd open my email and read a critical message and feel deflated. Then I'd get a great idea for a class I was preparing

and feel inspired. While reading the news, I'd feel consumed with worry about the world situation and with guilt because I'm not doing enough to heal it. Then a student would tell me how much I'd helped her and I'd feel worthy. As long as my sense of being is identified with what the yogic texts call the limited self, or false self, I'm going to go up and down.[1]

As I mentioned previously, ego is used very differently in yoga than in Western psychology. Sometimes the Sanskrit word *asmita* is defined as ego, but I think it's a little different. Asmita refers to identification with the part of us that is changing as opposed to the unchanging, permanent atman or spirit. It means "I-am-ness," and refers to the way the mind limits our unlimited consciousness.

Another Sanskrit term, *ahamkara*, is also translated as ego, and it has a slightly different meaning than asmita. It refers to the storyteller in our head, or the part of us that says, "I did that," "That's mine," or "Look at me!" It doesn't seem like we have clear terminology in English to reflect the detailed yogic understanding of the mind. It could be because in the West we are so completely identified with our minds. Yoga teaches us to identify with spirit and to understand that the mind is transitory and so is the body.

Just like so many others, I fell in love with asana when I was younger, and I would push myself into lots of contorted shapes. I got injured multiple times until finally, lying in pain, I realized that I wasn't actually doing yoga when I was practicing asana in a competitive, goal-oriented way. In the end it made me wonder, did I stumble on the very obstacles that Patanjali described so succinctly in his Yoga Sutras? Patanjali explains that because of our spiritual ignorance (avidya), we have an ego-mind that steps in to personalize everything, preventing us from seeing our true selves. In sutra 2.6 he says, "Ego (*asmita*) is (to consider) the nature of the seer and the nature of the instrumental power of seeing to be the same thing."[2] In other words, we've mistakenly equated mind with spirit. It's like the ego-mind has usurped the power of the spirit. It reminds me of this powerful poem by Rumi:

THE JAR WITH THE DRY RIM
The mind is an ocean . . . and so many worlds
Are rolling there, mysterious, dimly seen!

And our bodies? Our body is a cup, floating
On the ocean; soon it will fill, and sink. . . .
Not even one bubble will show where it went down.

The spirit is so near that you can't see it!
But reach for it . . . Don't be a jar
Full of water, whose rim is always dry.
Don't be the rider who gallops all night
And never sees the horse that is beneath him.[3]

The image of a jar with a dry rim floating on the ocean is very powerful. To me, the ocean represents spirit, the essence that permeates everything. Our body is the cup, seemingly independent and separate from the rest of creation, and from other people. But the water is inside and the water is outside. Spirit is us and all around us. "The spirit is so near that you can't see it!" Somehow we move through life with a dry rim, untouched by the spirit, the water we are literally swimming in. It's similar to the idea of not seeing your own eyes and a great analogy for asmita.

To be the rider who gallops all night and never sees the horse that is beneath him means that we are oblivious to the energy that animates us. This is a great example of ahamkara. Once again, our mind has somehow taken responsibility for the life that has been given to us. It's like a light bulb saying that it makes light. On the one hand that's true. Our mind is necessary to live. We need an ego to exist in the world. But, without electricity, a light bulb doesn't make light. Without spirit our mind wouldn't exist.

It reminds me of one night many years ago, when my son was very young, and I let him help me cook dinner. He was very proud of himself when all he had really done was make a big mess. I think I gave him a job like tearing up the lettuce, while I was running around doing everything—and cleaning up after him. When dinner was served, he proudly announced, "I made dinner!" It's sweet in a small child, but our minds are like children taking responsibility for things that we really have no responsibility for. Left unchecked, our ego-mind firmly establishes itself as the one who is responsible for all we do. According to Pandit Rajmani Tigunait, this ego-mind:

is a confused state of consciousness, unsure of its true identity. Its intentions and actions are smeared with confusion. As asmita (ego) matures, its belief in its distorted understanding of itself also matures, until it altogether overshadows the experience of our true nature. This is how a new reality—asmita—emerges from avidya (ignorance).[4]

## INDIVIDUALISM

Undoing this confusion is the work of a lifetime—or many lifetimes. The ego-mind is tricky and can even engage in spiritual practices without giving up one ounce of ownership of its sense of self. This is part of the reason I find it useful to go back to ancient texts rather than only studying with contemporary teachers. Personality can interfere with our experience of the truth. Even worse, the teachings can be distorted and used to control and abuse people.

Part of the problem is the capitalist concept of individualism that is built on the shaky foundation of personal achievement. We aren't trained to thank our ancestors for the sacrifices they made to get us where we are today. We don't want to see the invisible support of community, nature, and—most of all—spirit working through us tirelessly. We want to take responsibility for the good things that happen to us, and blame others when something goes wrong.

I recently watched a commercial for a large yoga clothing brand. It had the expected inspirational imagery with a relatively diverse group of people represented—although disabilities, large bodies, and seniors were not included. The ending message of the commercial was the brand's commitment to "everybody reaching their potential." The image that was associated with this phrase was someone standing proudly on a mountaintop alone, fist raised in the air. The celebration of this individual achievement, climbing to the mountaintop (because you were wearing the right outfit) felt off to me since it denies the communal nature of our existence, and of our yoga practice.

Something else about this imagery didn't sit well with me, and I wasn't sure why. It finally dawned on me that the potential they were talking about is the potential to climb that mountain—to overcome physical, exercise-oriented, obstacles—just like standing on your head or touching your toes. Is that the goal of yoga, or is that self-enhancement, an orientation that can lead to further confusion and deepens our ignorance? Research shows that spiritual training can lead to narcissism—even though it's really the antithesis of our goal.[5]

The next time you're taking a group yoga class, notice how much you think about the other students. Notice if your mind perceives the others as community or competition. Is the group class a format for communion with other practitioners or a stage for you either to show off or make yourself feel bad? These are all natural reactions, and they might shift from moment to moment, but it's helpful to bring awareness to the way the mind responds to others in a group yoga setting.

Much of the history of yoga is a tradition of asceticism—of transcending the body through force. "Hatha yoga" literally means "forceful yoga." If you want to do a traditional yoga practice you might want to consider holding one arm in the air for a few years or standing on one leg for a couple of months. Those are some of the ascetic practices that have been around for centuries and are still being practiced today.

## WHY AM I PRACTICING?

But there is a subtler theme in the history of yoga: a theme of overcoming egoism and selfishness through service and love. Bhakti yoga, the yoga of devotion; jnana yoga, the yoga of wisdom; and karma yoga, the yoga of selfless action, all teach us another way. They teach us that reaching our potential can only come when we transcend our own selfishness and allow our lives to become a vehicle for the energy and wisdom of the universe to flow through us. The question is: Can we allow yoga to help us transmute the energy of the ego-mind into service, or are we too tangled in spandex?

Service can be a confusing concept, because it's often wrongly defined as volunteering. While I think all yoga teachers should be paid for their work (after all we need to eat too), we can still offer our teaching as service. Service is really about seeing ourselves in others and acting from a place of love and compassion, rather than doing it for our ego-mind.

Another way to understand service is to think of it as connection. To focus on the collective is to raise our awareness above the ego-mind and to be with others. Some people are naturally service-oriented and nurturing, and often they're not supported by a culture that values ego-driven success. To move against this cultural selfishness, it can be helpful to think of those people in your life who are focused on the collective and consider how you can support them.

Community is one of the great revelations of yoga practice. It's a dialectic. While yoga is an individual, inner practice, it's also about community. The energy of the group inspires us and supports us. In a group setting, meditation is contagious, and we can find a stillness that is elusive when we're on our own. The true healing power of yoga is unlocked in shared practice. Just as we have understood that the body is not separate from the mind, we need to learn that the individual is not separate from the collective. We know that isolation is deadly, and yoga literally brings us together. The question is: Can we connect with others in our heart?

Occasionally, it's important to stop and ask yourself: Why am I practicing? What is my goal? Then consider if your practice is taking you there. Of course, you can allow your "why" to evolve. If you started practicing for physical reasons—to reduce back pain, to get more flexible, or to get stronger—can you now allow yoga to expose the truth of your ego? Can your practice reveal the part of your mind telling you to do more, get more, and compete with others? Does the strength you find in a *vinyasa* flow translate into the power to discriminate between ego-mind and spirit? Can you allow your yoga and your relationship to your mind to evolve?

> Why did you start practicing yoga? Do you still practice for that reason, or has it changed? What brings you to the mat or to a yoga class? What keeps you away from the mat or a yoga class?

## YOGA COMMUNITY OR YOGA INDUSTRY

So much changes over the arc of time, and so much stays the same. Recent research has revealed that over the course of millions of years, five different animals have separately evolved into crabs.[6] Yes, you read that right: five different kinds of animals went through their own evolution and all ended up like crabs. It's astounding to consider that crabs are so effective and efficient evolutionarily that different animals have become crabs, or crab-like.

This research made me reflect on the human condition and our tendency to recreate unresolved issues in our personal lives: Don't we end up marrying someone just like one of our parents, or literally becoming our parents as we age? It seems like an unavoidable aspect of human nature is that we are destined to repeat our past mistakes. I wonder if there's something similar happening in the yoga world? I sure hope not. The history of yoga in the West provides too many examples of yoga empires built on manipulation and abuse. The most recent examples are Bikram, Ashtanga, Sivananda Vedanta, and Kundalini, which have all had major abuse scandals in the last few years.

Are we destined to repeat this history, or can we find another way forward post-COVID where we engage with our practice effectively enough to see through our samskaras (the mind's conditioned habits)? The question is: Can the demise of the modern yoga studio offer an opportunity to build something new in its place, or are we destined to recreate the same issues that plagued the industry before the pandemic? Those issues include a lack of accessibility, racism, abuse, and unaddressed cultural appropriation. These issues all stem from a system based on greed and profiteering, rather than a system built on the foundational yoga teachings.

In other words, the yoga industry became a hollow shell, serving up a form of practice divorced from the philosophical and moral foundations of the very thing it was purportedly selling. The yoga industry became a crab: it evolved into that same form that our greed and selfishness often recreate, a system built on profit and bottom lines.

## FIRST DO NO HARM

The core teachings of yoga offer a pathway to fulfillment by turning within, rather than looking outside for pleasure or power to fill us up. How can we reconcile a yoga community run by business interests trying to sell us something? Yoga marketing is usually based on aspiration: the idea that there's something wrong with us that we need to fix. This is the opposite of yoga philosophy that encourages us to remember the truth of our fullness, and implores us to reconnect with the joy in our own hearts.

So how do we build back better? How do we create a yoga *community* rather than a yoga *industry* based on profit? To be honest, we probably can't.

Is it inevitable that we're just going to build another crab? But there might be a group of us that breaks off and has a chance to evolve into something else—maybe a jellyfish, or an octopus? I imagine that commercial yoga will come roaring back at some point. I don't think we can stop that evolution, but we don't have to contribute to it.

We can create a different kind of yoga community built on yoga's foundational ethics: ahimsa, nonviolence and compassion, and satya, truthfulness, or honesty. This means we need to acknowledge the harm that has been done in the name of yoga and commit to change. It's not about shame, but clarity (viveka).

I'm not suggesting we create a new organization, new teacher-training standards, or a new yoga style. Instead, I am simply asking you, how can you become more dedicated to the truth of yoga in your life? (And I'm asking myself these same questions.) Is there a way to dedicate ourselves to the truth of yoga, rather than the lie of yoga marketing? If so, it starts with self-inquiry, asking ourselves questions about the nature of our practice.

> Am I dedicated to my own freedom? What would my practice look like if it were based on the goal of freedom for myself and others?

The work I do on myself contributes to the community because I create less harm in the world. I often think of the medical profession and their oath, "First do no harm" (Although that exact line doesn't appear in the Hippocratic Oath). My practice allows me to support myself and see my own mind and the way it works more clearly.

If we could begin our practice by considering the impact we are having on others, I think we could reduce much of the harm that occurs in the world. If we could be brave enough to see our own prejudices, our own racism, transphobia, and so forth, then we could act in small ways to dismantle the systems that create those harmful beliefs and the structures that support them. Or, if we at least admitted to our shortcomings, we could find teachers to help us see those internalized systems more clearly. Although, we have to choose our teachers wisely.

My practice also allows me to truly be of service to others by showing me how to fill up my own well, rather than constantly looking outward for others to validate or support me. I don't know about you, but I tend to spend a lot of energy looking for external validation. It can be the thrill of getting likes on a Facebook post or wanting a compliment for something I've done. My practice allows me to see the way my mind seeks fulfillment in the world.

I often think about the way I react to criticism and how sensitive my ego-mind can be. Why is one small criticism so much more powerful than lots of praise? Imagine you're a yoga teacher and you have five students in your class. As the students leave, each one makes a comment. The first four offer praise: "Nice class," "That was great," "Thanks for that," "I feel so much better." Then the last student shrugs, and says, "So-so," as they walk out the door. Which of those five students will you be thinking of hours later?

All of us can consider the way we are practicing and teaching yoga, and the impact we are having on the world around us. By going on this intimately personal exploration of our mind and the way we are engaged in the practice, we can find more peace for ourselves and help to create a more peaceful and just world. This inner work also allows us to come together in our hearts and create a yoga community that is actually based in yoga, with its moral foundation. Otherwise, we just end up evolving into crabs.

Notice your reaction to praise and blame. Does your mind rely on these external messages for your self-worth?

# 11 | ENGAGED YOGA

I'VE BEEN THINKING a lot about happy endings, and whether I'm an optimist or if I'm just in denial. I've been trained by Hollywood movies to believe that somehow everything will work out in the end: the couple will get back together, justice will be served, and the bad guy will get what's coming to him. I've been taught to expect plot twists and lots of tension to keep me glued to the screen, but I've seen enough movies to know it will all work out in the end.

Unfortunately, reality is different than movies. Innocent people go to jail, and guilty people go free. Bad things happen to good people. Yet, I often hear people in the yoga community use the teaching of karma as an excuse when we're faced with situations that don't follow our "happy endings" logic. If a bad thing happens to a good person, we can't simply explain it away by saying, "That's karma!" Instead, we need to be willing to look at structural issues that might have caused that situation.

In particular, we have to be careful to not use the teaching of karma to explain away systemic injustices like structural racism. Karma isn't simply what happens to us, it's also what we do. In fact, the confusion around the word *karma* often stems from the fact that the same word means action and the consequence of action. According to the teachings, karma is so complex that it is beyond our comprehension.

Patanjali explains that only when we have perfected the ethical practice of nonattachment, or non-greed, aparigraha, can we begin to see the interconnected web of karma. According to one translation of sutra 2.39 by the renowned writer Christopher Isherwood (a gay man who wrote the story for the musical *Cabaret* and later became a dedicated yoga practitioner) and his teacher, Swami Prabhavananda, "When a man becomes steadfast in his abstention from greed, he gains knowledge of his past, present, and future existences." They then offer this explanation of how our attachments keep us from the true knowledge of our karma:

Attachment, and the anxiety which accompanies attachment, are obstacles to knowledge. As long as you are clinging desperately to the face of a precipice (and thereby to your life) you are in no condition to survey the place you climbed up from or the place toward which you are climbing. So Patanjali tells us that freedom from attachment will result in knowledge of the whole course of our human journey, through past and future existences.[1]

The point is that because we are so confused by our attachments, and because of the complexity of karma, it's impossible for our mind to comprehend it all. That also means that it's not an excuse to explain away why things happened. If you have privilege in this life, you can't simply think, "I must have been good in a previous life," and ignore the fact that your privilege probably has more to do with proximity to power and resources.

Similar to privilege, the way that punishment is doled out in society isn't simply "karma." Instead, we find the influence of racism and other forms of oppression. For example, there is a clear connection between racism and the death penalty in America. According to the Death Penalty Information Center, "Racial bias against defendants of color and in favor of white victims has a strong effect on who is capitally prosecuted, sentenced to death, and executed."[2] In fact, research shows that the chance of a capital conviction increased seventeen times if the victim of the crime was white.[3]

Karma is so often used to explain away the past, but really the teaching of karma is a directive to engage us in ethical behavior in the present moment. As I mentioned earlier, karma is not just reaction, it's about action. Karma represents our agency in this moment, our creativity, personal expression, and liberation. Karma, as action, encapsulates the idea of personal choice (the very opposite of karma as punishment). In the end, the choices we make in every moment create our future. Maybe we have it backward—karma is really all about choice and power.

That is exactly what we've seen with the Black Lives Matter movement: people taking action against racism. BLM is the largest civil rights movement in history, and more people protested around the world than ever before, taking action and speaking up against all the insidious forms of racism.[4] At its heart, the movement is an expression of love for all those

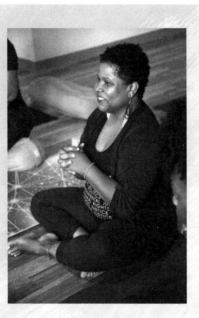

## OCTAVIA RAHEEM

My Ancestors didn't come here voluntarily. Until only a few decades ago, many didn't own their bodies or have access to basic freedoms. Despite that legacy of being physically bound and systemically shut out of so much, I know that my existence is evidence of their belief and faith that freedom was/is our birthright. For me yoga is a practice toward liberation. It is a space to examine and shed the chains that are not mine to carry. It is an opportunity to untangle myself from the traps, projections, narratives, and expectations that domi nant culture purports about people like me—a southern-born Black American woman.

Through my yoga practice I have learned how to access freedom in my body and breath, space in my mind and heart. I connect to the wisdom in my soul—wisdom forged across space and time by my ancestors.

"The function of freedom is to free someone else."—Toni Morrison who have been denied justice. As philosopher Cornel West said, "Never forget that justice is what love looks like in public."

This is the work that yoga demands of us—speaking out against injustice as an expression of ahimsa and love. This work is grounded in a holistic yoga practice that allows us to open our hearts with courage and compassion. In her groundbreaking book *Restorative Yoga for Ethnic and Race-Based Stress and Trauma*, Dr. Gail Parker explains:

> This is an inside job. The work I'm talking about is personal. We can begin the process ourselves. In order to effect social change, we have to approach the task of educating ourselves and of healing our internal wounds with courage, dedication, and devotion. But the work we have to do goes beyond policy changes, diversity and inclusion initiatives, and laws. The work we have to do requires shifts in consciousness and it starts with individual personal transformation. No law or policy can make that happen. It is time to shine a light on our own ethnic and racial wounds and to begin the process of healing ourselves. This new revolution is going to be internalized, not broadcast or televised. Now is a time for a change of heart, change that occurs from the inside out.[5]

## SOCIAL JUSTICE AS A PRACTICE

When George Floyd was murdered we saw a strong reaction in the yoga community. Many white yoga teachers started looking for ways to support Black Lives Matter. Some of it was very effective: there were educational campaigns, lists of Black teachers to follow, financial contributions to Black organizations, and some substantial efforts to shift culture. But some of it felt performative and simply offensive.

Engaging in social justice as a yoga practitioner doesn't mean you need to get involved with every movement, nor does it mean that you have to be an expert at social justice. What it means is that you see social justice as part of your yoga practice—something you *practice*, not something you perform or perfect. And it's an ongoing practice, not a onetime thing.

The most important step in practicing social justice is being open to learning. If you're not a member of a group directly impacted by a form of oppression, then you need to step back and listen and learn from people who are directly impacted. Even though you may be very energized and motivated to act, it doesn't mean you should. First, you need to do your own work. Look at the ways that you are personally participating in oppressing that particular group, whether consciously or unconsciously, directly or indirectly.

This is where your other yoga practices come in. Through asana, pranayama, and meditation, you build up resilience and strength to see yourself more clearly. You also build up the strength to be able to stand in the discomfort of the oppression that you may be creating in the world, or participating in. As I mentioned earlier, the Gita explains that the highest form of enlightenment is to see yourself in others. This doesn't mean that we pretend that everyone is having the same experience that we're having because "we're all one." It means that we are truly open to hearing, seeing, and feeling other people's suffering.

If you see harm being done to a marginalized person or community, you can educate yourself and do some research about the history of that marginalized group—Google is a great resource. You don't have to ask someone from that group to teach you, but if you do, make sure that you pay them for their time. Begin to make a connection between the experiences of other people and your own life. Look around you and see where you may have been ignorant about other people's suffering.

Finally, you can approach leaders who are already working in that area to listen and learn. For example, if you're not queer or trans, and you want to support the queer and trans community, it's not a good idea to create some programming about queer and trans issues or to start a new organization. Instead, do some research and find out who is already doing the work. There are already people from all marginalized groups working to free their communities from oppression. The best thing you can do is to ask them, "How can I be of service?"

If you're from a marginalized group, you can also do your research. Find other leaders to connect with, and know that you're not alone in the work. Community, *sangha* in Sanskrit, is the container for meaningful yoga practice, and the essence of social justice. Use the practices to build yourself up, to find strength, resilience, and joy, even in the midst of suffering. Living your life to its fullest is the most potent form of resistance for people who are oppressed.

## REFINE YOUR FOCUS

Perhaps the only thing we can control in life is the way we respond to internal and external stimuli. So the central consideration of our lives becomes a question of how we process information in this moment, and whether we decide to act, or not to act, based on the experience of that information. Essentially, the work of the yoga practitioner is to cultivate self-awareness and to unearth the mechanism behind this process. This reminds me of a quote attributed to Viktor Frankl, whom I mentioned earlier, "Between stimulus and response there is a space. In that space is our power to choose our response. In our response lies our growth and our freedom."[6]

The ability to create space is a skill we develop in our practice. Our asana, pranayama, and meditation all strengthen the ability to step back and observe how we function. With that skill, we can begin to consider the influences that affect the choices we make? Are these choices based on past experiences, personal preference, or the influence of others? We analyze the way we make decisions, and we make sure that our choices are based in ethics rather than based simply in our pursuit of personal fulfillment. We constantly ask ourselves if our actions and reactions are in alignment with nonviolence and truthfulness or based in selfishness. Are we acting with our heart at peace?

> Reflect on a recent decision that you made, something of importance in your life. How did you come to that decision? What process did you use to consider the pros and cons? Did you spend time considering the impact the choice had on you personally as well as the impact it had on others? Can you refine this process in some way?

One thing to consider when making big decisions is the role of emotion. As I discussed earlier regarding grief, all strong emotions have a powerful impact on the mind. These are like tidal-wave vrittis (thoughts) in the mind, knocking us over, and possibly leaving us confused and unable to think clearly. Have you ever made a bad choice from an emotional place? If I'm being honest, I see that anger, in particular, influences my ability to think clearly, and I sometimes find myself rewriting the past to defend myself when I'm in that state. Do you ever bicker with someone and say,

"No you said it like this . . ." and even as you're saying the words you know that what you're saying is not true, or at least greatly exaggerated to defend your position?

In a subtle form, this idea of personal choice can be understood as a question of where we put our attention. In yoga, the mind is linked to the energy or life force known as *prana*, so it's important to regulate how we use both. Do I focus my prana on spiritual awakening through service, or do I focus my prana on fulfilling my selfish desires? It's not that you need to be a saint. It's just that we have it all backwards. We think that happiness comes from getting what we want. But yoga shows us that happiness comes through service and that selfish desire is actually the source of our unhappiness.

The question of how we use our prana is also the challenge of brahmacharya, the fourth precept of yama, the first limb of ashtanga yoga. Traditionally, brahmacharya is the vow of celibacy that monks take. Celibacy was supposed to offer renunciants freedom from the worldly attachments of relationships. But we've clearly seen the damage that is so often done when people take vows of celibacy and end up as sexual abusers or being sexually inappropriate. The idea behind brahmacharya is that instead of focusing their energy on one primary relationship and immediate family, a monk can serve all and love all. In practice, brahmacharya isn't specifically about not having sex, rather it's about making conscious decisions about where we focus our energy. In relationships, brahmacharya can represent healthy boundaries as we learn to respect our partners and practice ahimsa, non-harming.

Instead of simply denying our sexuality, brahmacharya, and similarly karma, are questions of focus and attention. Are we focused on the well-being of ourselves, our loved ones, our community, or the world at large? This expands to questions about our role in the world and whether it's okay to just sit back and watch the world go by, or whether we should be speaking up and acting. It's a question of whether we should only be focused on the fulfillment of our own desires, or if we recognize that our happiness is intimately linked to the happiness of others. There is a beautiful line in the Gita that speaks to this question of personal desire, and whether we can see the interconnectedness of all our individual desires. In the end, all these small desires are fragments of a deeper yearning for spiritual connection and peace.

Someone with personal desires will not experience true peace. But when all desires merge, like different rivers flowing into the vast, deep ocean, then peace is easily realized.[7]

## ACTION AND INACTION

Once again, this question of whether and how to act reminds me of the situation that Arjuna finds himself in: an epic battle between good and evil. Honestly, I feel for Arjuna because I usually don't feel like fighting either. But you can't deny the parallel between Arjuna's plight and ours. The quest to understand our role in the world is a universal conundrum that we all find ourselves in. And that is the question the Gita answers: Our dharma is the service we are destined to perform.

Also, it would be easy to say that Krishna is emboldening us to fight against evil and stand up for justice. I could make the obvious parallel between Arjuna's battle and our contemporary fight for social justice. But we have to be careful about using ancient scripture to justify our actions in the present day. God knows, the Bible has been misused to manipulate us and convince us that we should act in certain ways that the church wants us to.

The German philosopher Friedrich Nietzsche explained that the whole concept of good and evil was created by the Catholic Church to control people's behavior.[8] It's amazing to consider the ways that language and culture are used to control us. To think that the concepts of evil—and hell—were created to keep us in line is horrific because they have such powerful real-life consequences. I know many queer people who have been outcast from their families because of the power of the lie that being queer is somehow evil.

Instead of simply saying that Krishna is telling us to stand up for social justice and fight our just war, we can look at the teaching for what it is: a challenge to find our inner warrior. The teachings are about the battle raging between our own heart and mind, an inner conflict. Our job is to listen to the song (*gita*) of our own heart. Does that song express itself in the alignment of our thoughts, words, and deeds? Or do we continue to pursue the fulfillment of our selfish desires?

At one point, Krishna explains to Arjuna that none of us really have a choice between acting or not acting. We are always acting, always doing something. So rather than pretending that we're sitting back and observing, we have to realize that we are always making decisions and taking action in every moment. Krishna explains:

> Ceasing to do things will not make you "actionless." Nor will you rise to perfection simply by renouncing actions.
>
> No one is free of actions even for a moment, because everyone is moved to do things by the qualities of nature.
>
> Do your duty; such action is better than doing nothing. If you attempt to renounce all actions, it would be impossible to maintain your body.
>
> The world is bondage when actions are done just for your own sake. Therefore, Arjuna, make every action a sacrifice, utterly free of personal attachment.[9]

Krishna's message is that we can't simply stop acting. We are making choices in every moment that affect our lives and the lives of those around us. This reminds me of how so many people say they aren't interested in politics and don't vote. In the 2016 U.S. election, millions of people didn't vote because they thought Clinton would easily win, or maybe because they didn't really care. That act of not voting contributed to Trump winning, and the degradation of rights for marginalized people in the United States over the course of his presidency.

The point is, when you don't act you actually *do* make a very strong statement. If you don't speak up when you hear a racist or homophobic comment you are still acting, and condoning that behavior. I'm not saying you have to go out and fight on the street or join political demonstrations, but you have to act. You have to act and take responsibility for this moment and how your actions will contribute to it one way or another. Your actions can contribute to greater division and more inequity, or you can stand up, act, and speak out for righteousness.

The term *dharma* is used to refer to this personal focus for your life and the way you use your energy. I often wonder about my identity as an activist and also as a teacher. I spent many years demonstrating, disrupting systems, and getting arrested for it. I've also spent many years teaching and trying to build community. I see both efforts as my dharma. Tearing down deadly and destructive systems is also a creative way to build something new.

Consider the focus of your dharma. One clue is simply paying attention to what fills your thoughts. Do you spend a lot of time thinking about your children, your job, your activism? Whatever you are focusing the majority of your energy on is your dharma. If you are disabled, and you spend a lot of time focusing on caring for yourself, that is your dharma. One person's dharma is not better or worse than someone else's, but it can be helpful to be clear about where you are focusing your attention.

## YOGA OFF THE MAT

The other day I posted a quote by Lakshmi Nair on my Instagram feed that read, "A yoga that doesn't hold social justice at its heart is not a complete or true yoga." Lakshmi is a powerful voice in the yoga and social justice movement, and the creator of the Satya Yoga Cooperative in Denver, Colorado, which is one of the first yoga cooperatives for people of color in the United States. The next morning, I woke up to a comment on the post that really got my attention. Someone had replied that people don't come to yoga to hear about social justice, and that yoga teachers should stay in their lane and not talk about things they don't know about.

We only need to look back to Gandhi to see the connection between yoga and social justice. He explained:

> But this much I can say with assurance, as a result of all my experiments, that a perfect vision of Truth can only follow a complete realization of *Ahimsa*. To see the universal and all-pervading Spirit of Truth face to face one must be able to love the meanest of creation as oneself. And a man who aspires after that cannot afford to keep out of any field of life. That is why my devotion to Truth has drawn me into the field of politics; and I can say without the slightest hesitation, and yet in all humility, that those who say that religion has nothing to do with politics do not know what religion means. Identification with everything that lives is impossible without self-purification; without self-purification the observance of the law of *Ahimsa* must remain an empty dream; God can never be realized by one who is not pure of heart."[10]

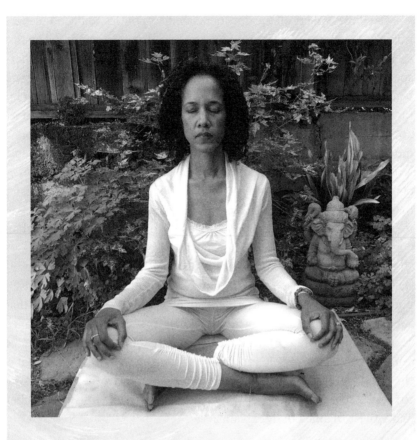

### KAMALA ITZEL HAYWARD

My practice is to work toward creating a world where all living beings are seen as divine—where all people have access to the resources, opportunities, and privileges they need to experience safety, well-being, and freedom from oppression. In other words, I see my social justice work as my primary yoga practice. And while this work certainly benefits me as a being in this world, I hold it largely as selfless service. I'm trying to help shape a direction toward a destination that we may not reach until long after this lifetime.

Gandhi connects all the dots here: ahimsa, politics, and God realization. Yet I realize that this misunderstanding, that yoga and social justice aren't related, is probably very common in our community. Yoga teachers spend the vast majority of their time and training focused on learning and teaching asana. They may receive a short training in yoga history and philosophy, but I wonder about the quality and depth of that portion of most 200-hour yoga teacher trainings. I imagine that most of those philosophy modules are not focused on the ways that contemporary yoga is so deeply intertwined with social justice. To me, the most important point is to recognize that just because yoga is taught as asana most of the time doesn't make that correct or true. This is basic cultural appropriation—settling for a whittled-down version of the expansive yoga teachings—rather than being willing to explore their depth and mind-bending truths.

As we've been discussing, yoga is a spiritual practice dedicated to transcending the limited aspects of the mind and opening the heart. It's a discipline designed to remove suffering—our own as well as the suffering that we experience around us. Yoga teaches us how to see beyond the ignorance of our myopic self-importance so that we can experience the grandeur of our interconnectedness. It's about seeing myself in you. In a sense, that is the definition of social justice, seeing ourselves in each other and working to create a society where all people are treated fairly and justly. As teacher and activist Dianne Bondy explains:

> We are missing a huge piece of what the yoga practice is intended to be. The yoga community, and more detrimentally the yoga industry as a whole, is missing the pinnacle niyama—svadhyaya, or self-study. Collectively, we are not practicing or celebrating the act of self-reflection and compassion that is self-study. Too many of us fail to acknowledge our biases, privileges, and limiting beliefs.[11]

Yoga begins when we step back from our own assumptions and begin to question our thinking, our attachments, and our cultural conditioning. Yoga creates space in our body, our breath, and our mind to allow for truth to emerge. When we relax the body and quiet the mind, our heart steps forward to speak the truth. We experience the power of that truth, satya, in directing our actions. We can ask ourselves how we have contributed to, or silently supported, a culture based on white supremacy. We can ask ourselves how we may be overtly or covertly racist, ableist, or homophobic.

As we consider how to move forward in a world that seems chaotic, where there is hatred, evil, and selfishness, yoga shows us the way. Yoga doesn't offer a simple answer to resolve our political conflicts, but it shows the way—and it's a way inward to connect with truth and love in our own heart. With that strong inner connection, we can practice social justice—service in action—to create a world that reflects yoga's message of unity, equity, and justice.

## 12 | BUILDING COMMUNITY

IN 2013, MY HUSBAND Matt and I decided to move our family to Santa Barbara from the San Francisco Bay Area where we'd been living for over twenty years. I struggled with leaving my yoga community, which I had been nurtured by for so long. It was especially hard to leave all of my students whom I felt very dedicated to. I also dreaded starting my yoga teaching career all over again in a new town. As teachers, we have to be experts at so many different things—marketing, accounting, and yoga! After building a yoga community for so long it was hard to just let it all go.

When I moved here I found myself lost and confused about how to proceed. I didn't have a community, and I began to see how important it was for me to have the support of other yoga practitioners, both for my own personal practice as well as for my teaching. I knew one yoga teacher in Santa Barbara, Cheri Clampett, and she was teaching yoga to people with cancer at the local hospital. I found myself getting envious of her work, which seemed like a really strange reaction to have when someone is doing something so wonderful.

I was struggling and jealous, so I decided I should practice what I preach and try to use the yoga practices to help process my feelings. So I thought about how I could apply the teaching of *pratipaksha bhavana* to the situation, because I saw how my thinking was causing me pain. Remember, that teaching is about positive thinking, cultivating the opposite thought, or reflecting on the outcome of negative thinking.

That practice made me realize that I could turn the situation around by supporting Cheri and lifting her up, rather than allowing myself to be deluded by my ego's selfishness. As I was sitting in meditation, thinking about this, I had an image come to me of Cheri standing on a stage teaching. That is what led me to the idea of creating the Accessible Yoga Conference. I thought I could simultaneously support my friend and try to build the community that I was seeking—a mutually supportive yoga community dedicated to the ideals of accessibility and equity. A few months later, we had the first conference in Santa Barbara, and Cheri was one of the presenters. It was a lesson to me in the power of the teachings and the fact that my ego doesn't always know what's best for me. It also showed me how one selfless thought can change my life.

The American ideal of rugged individualism is at odds with yoga philosophy—and with logic. While yoga is a completely personal practice, it only happens in community. Our practice is built on the support of our friends, teachers, students, and the wisdom of our yoga ancestors. After that experience with the conference, I realized that the focus on building up my own teaching practice was too limited. I shifted my focus to supporting other yoga teachers and creating a platform for their teaching. The main lesson for me was that I need to be vigilant in watching for the way my ego attaches to every situation. I've tried to avoid competition with other teachers by actively working to support them, which has allowed me to build a community outside the commercial yoga industry.

It seems contrary to logic, and the way we are usually trained, but if we are going to call ourselves yoga practitioners we need to bring yoga into all aspects of our lives, including business. Currently, this is the form my practice takes: avoid the trap of capitalism, and instead practice nonattachment and service to the best of my ability.

Can you think of someone you may be envious of? What is at the heart of that feeling? Is there a quality that you admire in that person? How could you cultivate that quality in yourself?

## COLLABORATION AS A PRACTICE

At every Accessible Yoga Conference, I give all the attendees the same homework assignment. I ask them to find someone at the conference they can support. This support can take many forms: for example, a collaboration of some kind, a networking lead, sharing about the other person's work on social media, and so much more. These individual efforts are the building blocks of a strong grassroots movement, and I've seen incredible connections come out of the conferences—whole organizations have been launched through these connections.

In the yoga world, we have a choice to support other people and organizations who are engaging in the practice in a way that resonates with us. It's not that large corporate yoga chains aren't made up of wonderful people trying to do the right thing. It's a question of voting with our dollars, and with our energy, to build a community that is a reflection of the yoga teachings themselves.

Sometimes it's hard to see how our individual actions impact the larger community. We tend to think that we live in our own little bubble and that no one is paying attention to what we do. But it's not true. Our actions can have a major impact on others. We can be an example of how to be in the world—or an example of how not to be!

One of the best practices for building community is to work collaboratively with other teachers and community members. Collaboration demands a certain amount of humility, and humility is antithetical to capitalism. It can take a refined eye to see the difference between humility and giving up power, but it's an essential difference. To put it simply, humility isn't giving up power to someone else. It's about having a realistic sense of ourselves. When we clearly see ourselves—our strengths and weaknesses—then we can enter into balanced relationships with others.

For a community to grow and flourish, its members must be gaining benefit from the group, and even better, the entire world is gaining some benefit. A strong community is offering service in the world and supporting its members in the process. In other words, the most effective communities are built on a foundation of service to their members and to the world at large.

This doesn't have to take the form of an organization, or some kind of formal structure. If you're an experienced teacher, or community leader, mentoring others is a great way to give back to your community. As leaders, we always have to focus on sharing power and training other people to take over our work. It's another powerful exercise in humility to constantly work on becoming irrelevant, which takes the focus away from individuals and puts it back on the mission at hand.

## SUPPORT MARGINALIZED STUDENTS AND TEACHERS

Yoga culture is not divorced from culture in general. We can see the ways that white supremacy has impacted contemporary yoga practice. We've idealized a certain body type and physical ability over all else. So many people are left out and excluded from the practice. While there has been a major shift over the past few years, there is still so much work to do. Yoga spaces need to be welcoming to anyone who is interested in practicing, and just because *you* feel welcome in a space doesn't mean other people do.

To successfully build community, we need to focus on the most marginalized individuals and make sure their needs are being met. Not only is this the way to create spaces that are truly welcoming but also members of the community who have privilege will benefit from learning how to make space for others. We see this in research on integrated school classrooms. When we stop segregating children with disabilities, and offer integrated learning spaces, everyone benefits, including disabled and nondisabled kids.[1]

The best way to diversify yoga spaces is to have those spaces led by a diverse group of people. For example, if you want Black people to come to yoga, support Black yoga teachers. It's very simple: supporting marginalized yoga teachers is the most effective way to create diverse yoga classes and to expand opportunities for marginalized students.

Also, we all learn from each other's diverse experiences, and I would suggest that marginalized teachers offer a different, and essential, perspective on the teachings. Shockingly, one of the most marginalized groups of yoga teachers in contemporary yoga are South Asian teachers. This is clearly the result of colonialism and cultural appropriation, which I'll discuss later. Many of these teachers have a direct connection to the teachings through culture and family, and are a precious resource for the yoga community at large.

## WHEN WE FEEL SAFE WE CAN RELAX

In order to cultivate a safe and supportive yoga community we need to start by looking at larger cultural issues that influence us, either consciously or unconsciously. We can also consider how to create spaces that foster inner connection and create a safe container that allows people to turn inward.

Ironically, our ability to turn within is often limited by our external experiences and lack of access to supportive environments for learning and growth. Most yoga spaces feel exclusive and unwelcoming to many people who are actively seeking support. We often talk about creating safe spaces, which refers to the idea that we can create spaces that are safe for people with marginalized identities.

But the question of whether a space is safe or not is a completely personal thing. Just because you intend to create a safe space doesn't mean that everyone will feel safe there. Even if a space feels safe to you, it may not work for someone else. That might be because they've experienced acute trauma or trauma based on a marginalized identity, such as racism, homophobia, or transphobia. Or, your efforts might be based solely on your experience, and someone else's trauma is different than yours.

On the other hand, the idea of a brave space[2] means that we're brave enough to address the issues that make people feel unsafe. It means we're willing to stop avoiding addressing prejudice, oppression, and white supremacy that interfere with the possibility of creating a container for all participants to make that inward journey. I realize that a yoga class may not seem like the place to have a hard conversation about race or gender. But I actually think there are many ways to allow for discussion and questioning to happen, whether it's before, during, or after class, or if it's in your social media posts.

Sure, it's easy to say "be inclusive," but that is really an outdated concept. We can't simply build an exclusive community and then invite marginalized people to join us after the fact. A welcoming community needs to be built on a foundation of safety and equity for all of its members, from the very beginning. In the end, the relative safety of a space directly affects the students' experience. Over the years, I've found that there are a number of factors that support students in allowing themselves to relax. In Shavasana in particular, you can see how safety is the most important factor, but lighting, temperature, and quiet are all essential elements that contribute to letting go.

Mei Lai Swan trains yoga teachers in trauma-informed teaching. She shares her thinking about the ways that yoga can become a source for personal healing, if we approach it correctly. Remember, safety is in the eye of the beholder. If you're a teacher, some ways that you can create safety in yoga spaces is through trauma-informed practices, which include not touching students without consent, offering choices in all practices—including opting out—and generally giving students a sense of agency and control of their body and their practice. Also, you have to be careful

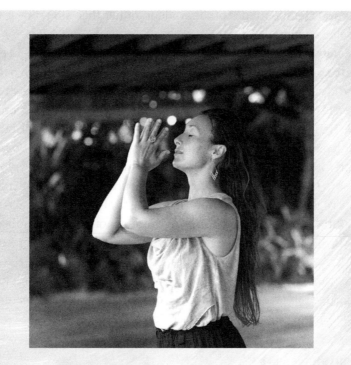

## MEI LAI SWAN

For me, yoga is not just in support of, but is at the heart of, my service and social justice work. In my late teens, I had some profound experiences of interconnectedness and compassion through the practices of meditation and yoga. These experiences birthed a deep fire to be of service through love, to care deeply for each other and our earth. This shifted me from studying astrophysics to a twenty-plus-year path of service through spiritual practice and teaching, community, and social justice work. These threads have eventually woven together into what I share today: embodied trauma-informed yoga and social justice education. My own practice has been both the fire and the water throughout. It has been a path of great personal transformation and healing, and has nourished me along the way with inner guidance, resilience, courage, and a strong ethical foundation. Yoga is truly my ground, my compass, my service, and my joy.

to respect the experience of the student, rather than assuming it will be the same as yours.

Safety is the key to letting go and resting. Most of us are taught that we have to constantly push ourselves to be productive and to earn our keep. These ideas are so engrained in us that we don't see the ways that stress has degraded our health, self-esteem, and the quality of our lives. According to Tricia Hersey, founder of the Nap Ministry, "Rest is a form of resistance because it pushes back against capitalism and white supremacy."[3] Yoga offers an antidote to the "go, go, go!" mentality of our lives, but not everyone has access to these life-changing and lifesaving practices. Our challenge is to create yoga spaces that are truly welcoming to all. But it demands that we are both generous and humble. It's worth asking yourself if you are hoarding yoga, in the same way you might hoard money, power, and other resources.

> What helps you to relax? The next time you practice meditation, guided relaxation, or restorative yoga make an effort to create an environment that will be conducive to truly letting go.

## SHARING POWER

This may be obvious, but community building is done through sharing power with people—power over their bodies and over their lives. This is where community building is distinguished from building a brand, having a following, or a starting a cult. A yoga "community" is defined by the fact that people are participating joyfully, and their participation is giving them more options, more power, and more agency in their lives. Giving people agency over their bodies and their lives means that if we are in a position of authority, we learn how to share power. It's normal to crave control, and for many of us it's an experience we rarely have. So in a yoga setting there may be a tendency to enforce a certain kind of behavior that is parallel to the cultural conditioning we can't seem to escape.

I remember when I started teaching yoga, one of the things I found most challenging was the occasional student who wouldn't follow along with the group and would completely do their own thing. I was confused about why someone would come to a yoga class and not do what everyone else was doing. My first reaction was to tell them to get in line, until I realized that my effort to control them stemmed from my own insecurities as a teacher, and as a person in general.

I struggled with the authority I had when leading a class. As a gay man, I had survived in a straight world by blending in and hiding in the shadows. It was a revelation to me to realize one day that my painful shyness was simply an out-of-control ego. I used to think that egotistical people were always loud and attention seeking, but, as I mentioned, that shyness is also a manifestation of ego. Once I realized that my interest in controlling my students was based on my own insecurities, I was able to stop. I released myself from the iron grip of their approval, and simultaneously, I released them from the grip of my approval.

I often wonder about the way we segregate people by level in yoga classes. Levels aren't reflective of the essence of the yoga teachings. I understand that students who have been practicing for many years may not want to be in the same class as brand-new students. But just because someone is extremely flexible, and can contort their body into shapes, doesn't make them an advanced yoga practitioner. The way we judge people by their level of strength and flexibility feels anathema to the underlying teachings of yoga.

Is there a way to shift our thinking away from the levels we use in yoga to some other benefit-based system? For example, what if we advertised, "Yoga for Strength" or "Yoga for Mobility" instead of "Advanced" and "Beginner"? There's nothing more beautiful than a yoga class filled with a diversity of students of all ages and abilities united by their breath, their inner focus, and their love of yoga. I actually think a diverse class can teach us all a lot more about the heart of yoga than a class where everyone is doing the exact same thing.

## THE POWER OF LANGUAGE

A good example of power dynamics is the way we use language and how sensitive, or insensitive, we are to the needs of others when we're speaking with them. This is especially clear in the terms we use to identify people. For example, within the disability community, there is a lot of discussion about language. There is currently some disagreement between the use of identity-first and person-first language that reflects the role of language in sharing power.

Person-first language means you would say, "a person with a disability," like "a person with Parkinson's disease." Identity-first language means you would say the identity first, such as, "an autistic person," or "a Blind person," or "a Deaf person." And actually, for many communities, specifically the autism, Deaf, and Blind communities, people generally prefer identity-first language, because they feel like their disability is an important part of their identity, and there's pride in that. Similarly, for BIPOC (Black, Indigenous, and People of Color), the power to decide how to refer to oneself is essential and will differ from person to person.

Pride is a way marginalized groups take back power. I remember marching with Queer Nation, an activist group in the 1990s. The main goal of that group was to empower queer people by raising awareness of our existence and need for basic human rights through language, imagery, and representation. We put posters and stickers everywhere, we made T-shirts and buttons with pro-queer slogans like, "Queer Nation: get used to it," or "Stop the violence: queers fight back!" Most importantly, we started a conversation about queer rights, and the way we took back the word *queer* was an important first step. It's now part of normal usage, but not long ago it was only used as a slur.

The point is that we don't get to decide what language other people use for their own identity. We have to be sensitive to people's preferences and ask them about it directly. Similarly, the correct use of pronouns is an essential way to respect someone's agency and authority over their body and their life. So, another way to make our spaces welcoming is to focus on gender as a spectrum and move away from the strict binary of male and female—gender essentialism.

There is a well-known character in the Mahabharata (the epic tale that includes the Gita) called Shikhandi, who is transgender.[4] Shikhandi was born as a woman but identified as a man and became a central figure in the famous battle that is the focus of the Gita's narrative. During the battle, Krishna defends Shikhandi's right to choose their gender as opposed to being stuck with the gender they were assigned at birth.

Let's take a cue from Krishna and respect people's gender identity and pronouns. In other words, you don't get to look at someone and decide, "You look male, therefore, I'll use he/him pronouns for you." Rather, you get to ask someone, "What pronouns do you use?" And even better than that, share your own pronouns when you introduce yourself. When I speak with people, and especially when I'm teaching, I try to introduce myself with my pronouns so that people know that it's safe for them to share their pronouns with me. I say, "Hi, my name is Jivana Heyman, and my pronouns are he/him."

The more we all speak about the use of pronouns publicly, especially people who hold space like yoga teachers, we can start to normalize the use of different pronouns and create safer spaces for trans and nonbinary folks. Normalizing the use of "they/them" as personal pronouns is another way that nonbinary folks feel seen and respected.

Avoiding the use of stereotypes in general is also important, and although I think we all try to avoid stereotyping each other, it still happens frequently. For example, teachers often assume the gender of a group of students because they appear to look a certain way. It's surprising how many times I've heard ridiculous stereotypes in yoga class. Often these are based on race, gender, or sexuality, but any kind of assumption is not helpful in terms of creating a welcoming space.

Beliefs about weight are some of the most pervasive and dangerous stereotypes in the yoga world. There's a lot of diet talk in yoga, and it is really not appropriate. Generally speaking, yoga teachers aren't trained as nutritionists and don't have any reason to discuss diet with students. Our first focus needs to be questioning our own ableist ideas about weight and health.

The fat pride movement is similar to the other civil rights movements. In fact, you can think of the word *fat* like *queer* and *disabled*. These are descriptive terms that communities are taking back with pride. One important step is that we need to stop assuming that fat people want to lose weight, which is a really offensive stereotype and another way that fat-phobia seeps into yoga.

With this awareness we can create a practice that is welcoming for fat yoga practitioners and offers an opportunity for self-care and empowerment. As Marc Settembrino shares in the sidebar, yoga was a gateway to their activism in the fat liberation movement, and it continues to sustain their activism.

## REACHING OUT

These issues can also be addressed in your marketing and the way you present yourself to the world. This includes the images you put in your marketing campaigns, images you have at your studio on flyers or on posters,

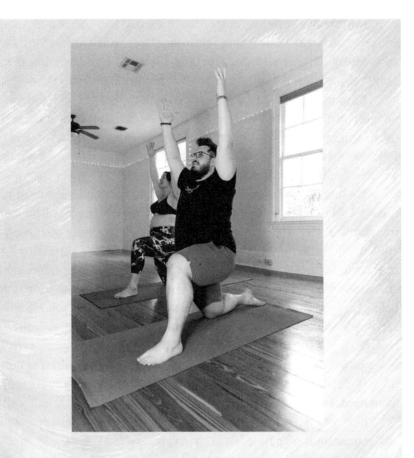

## MARC SETTEMBRINO

Practicing yoga (asana) empowered me to make peace with my body and understand that I am worthy of dignity, love, and acceptance just as I am. Today, most of my work as a yoga instructor centers on holding space for people in larger bodies to experience joyful movement and celebrate their bodies. Because fat bodies are objectified in our society, it's important for fat folks like me to reclaim our agency and bodies. We don't have these physical forms for very long, and you can't live fully if you are constantly waging war against your body. Yoga was my gateway into the fat liberation movement. So in a lot of ways my yoga practice both created and sustains my activism.

quotes that hang on the walls, and the posts you share on social media. Diversity is especially important in the way we represent what a yoga practitioner looks like. Also, in your marketing, ask yourself if you're speaking about people in a way that's welcoming and accessible. Repeating the slogan, "yoga for all" isn't enough, and the ideals of diversity and equity need to permeate through all the ways that you speak about and practice yoga.

I've noticed the hashtag #accessibleyoga has been used over 90,000 times on Instagram, which is very exciting. However, many teachers and brands are using #accessibleyoga without really understanding what it means. Simply saying, "yoga is accessible to anyone who wants to practice" isn't enough. It reflects an ignorance of the way that oppression works. Simply calling a class "Accessible Yoga" at the local yoga studio may not work either since many people may not feel welcome there. We need to look more deeply at all the ways we hold and share power.

Ask yourself, "Is the practice I'm offering truly accessible to all levels of practitioner?" If you are trying to make your classes as accessible as possible for people with disabilities, it's worth considering universal design. This is a holistic approach to accessibility that considers all aspects of people's lives, where they live, what their scheduling needs may be, what transportation options exist, and so on.

## SPIRITUAL BYPASSING

Spiritual bypassing is a term that is used to describe the way spiritual teachings are often used to avoid the difficult and painful aspects of life—in particular, painful emotions. It often takes the form of overly positive, uplifting, and inspiring messages that deny the pain that someone is experiencing, including ourselves. This form of bypassing encourages us to deny our true feelings. It leads us to the conclusion that painful or "negative" emotions or thoughts are less meaningful or less worthy than other kinds of emotions or thoughts.

Generally, I think a lot of spiritual bypassing happens by accident. We mean well and want to focus on the positive, and mostly we want other people to be happy as well. But by bypassing we are actually causing more harm. For example, we tend to talk about the positive transformational aspects of yoga without discussing the fact that our journey can, and usually is, a struggle. Yoga will unearth painful feelings—that's part of the practice. So someone's journey in yoga may not be all positive. They might have painful emotions arise during a practice, they might get injured, they might realize they've hurt other people. Guilt, shame, remorse, depression, and anxiety are the most powerful teachers we have. Although we don't need to seek them out, these emotions are precious too.

According to the psychotherapist John Welwood, who coined the phrase, spiritual bypassing occurs when we use, "Spiritual ideas and practices to sidestep personal, emotional 'unfinished business,' to shore up a shaky sense of self, or to belittle basic needs, feelings, and developmental tasks."[5] A large part of yoga is accepting every part of ourselves and becoming more of an integrated whole. In order to be integrated, we have to accept the pleasant and the painful, the positive and the negative.

As a holder of space, or as a teacher, we need to be aware of the importance of painful emotions and experiences for our students. We have to be careful to not create an environment that shames people or makes people feel less than if they have a negative reaction to something or if they have pain or difficult emotions arise. Somehow these painful emotions are only allowed to surface when we're practicing hip opening poses! Or at least that's what you'd surmise by attending many contemporary yoga classes. To be honest, I would just be more neutral about it and explain that we never know what will arise. Joy may arise and grief may arise. Any range of human emotion can arise for you, and that's okay.

I remember the second yoga class I ever taught. There was a woman practicing in the very front of the class. The minute I started teaching she lay down on her mat and started crying quietly. She spent the entire class crying. I was in a panicked state since it was my second yoga class ever, and I didn't know what to do with her. I completely ignored her. After class she came up to me and said, "Thank you so much for letting me be here and cry. I just needed a safe place." If I was more comfortable, I would have approached her during class and asked if there was anything I could do to support her. But in the end, just letting her be was actually the best choice.

So one of the things that can happen in yoga practice is that you become more sensitive. Increasing your sensitivity is a very positive thing, but it can actually lead to more suffering. It can make you feel the suffering of others as your own, which we've discussed earlier from the Bhagavad Gita when

Krishna explains that the highest form of enlightenment is compassion. I'll share a different translation of this beautiful passage here:

> As your mind becomes harmonized through yoga practices, you begin to see the *Atman* in all beings and all beings in your Self; you see the same Self everywhere and in everything.
>
> Those who see me wherever they look and recognize everything as my manifestation, never again feel separate from me, nor I from them.
>
> Whoever becomes established in the all-pervading oneness [of *Brahman*] and worships me abiding in all beings—however he may be living, that yogi lives in me.
>
> The yogi who perceives the essential oneness everywhere naturally feels the pleasure or pain of others as his or her own.[6]

Spiritual bypassing is the opposite of compassion. When we're bypassing, we focus on the positive only, or jump to the ideals of non-duality instead of acknowledging the duality of our distinct experiences. Saying, "we're all one" or "I don't see color" is a way to deny the pain of other people's lived experiences. Accepting the spectrum of other people's experience, and not judging them as good or bad, is the most effective way of creating a welcoming space and building a community.

# SUMMARY OF PART TWO

I REALIZE THAT writing a book about yoga and saying that it somehow can change the world may seem a little far-fetched. I'm not suggesting that practicing modern postural yoga necessarily creates social justice in the world. What I'm saying is that the philosophy of this practice is based in equity and justice. Revolutionary yoga is about seeing ourselves in others and living a life of service. These two elements—which I'm summarizing as courage and compassion—really can change the world.

Contrary to popular opinion, a yoga practitioner isn't always peaceful and unemotional. Part of the courage that yoga brings is the courage to engage with our emotions in an effective way. Anger can also be based in love and compassion. Expressed skillfully, righteous anger is the ethical response to witnessing someone causing harm. This is the result of compassion. If you feel the pain of another, then it's natural that you would feel anger when they are being injured—especially if they are being bullied or oppressed. This type of anger gets the mind's attention so we can respond appropriately, which could mean speaking out or defending the one who is being harmed. According to Gandhi:

> Use your anger for good. Anger to people is like gas to the automobile—it fuels you to move forward and get to a better place. Without it, we would not be motivated to rise to a challenge. It is an energy that compels us to define what is just and unjust.[1]

We need to be careful about trying to control our emotions in yoga. Instead, our emotions should be experienced—even appreciated and embraced. The energy of our emotions is the vehicle that our heart is using to express itself. You could even say that emotions are the language of the spirit, sending us messages from a deep part of ourselves beyond the mind. Embrace those messages.

This doesn't mean we act on our feelings. We can completely embrace our emotions, and then use our practices to come back to balance so that we act in conscious and conscientious ways. The process works like this: We see harm happening in the world, we have an emotional reaction and process those feelings. That means we feel whatever is coming up without acting on it. But, we pay attention because our emotions carry important messages. And we follow up with a question: How can my response contribute to reducing harm and suffering in the world?

In this way, we cultivate ahimsa by focusing on service. Our service is embodied compassion. Service demands that we get our personal motives out of the way and do our best to be present to the needs of those around us. Can our actions, our very lives, be offerings—dedicated service to our own sacred heart and to the heart of all humanity?

With this in mind, I'd like to take a moment to address yoga teachers, who are so often the public face of yoga. When we put ourselves out into the world as teachers, we become responsible for carrying the torch of yoga and passing it down to future generations. In order to do so, we need to consider how we can lift up the teachings now, at this moment in time. To that end, I worked with my team at Accessible Yoga to put together some suggestions in the form of a manifesto for yoga teachers. This summarizes the topics I've tried to address in the second part of the book:

ACCESSIBLE YOGA MANIFESTO

We believe yoga begins with ahimsa: non-harm and compassion for all. This means disrupting systems of oppression and calling out harm when we see it.

We believe in recognizing each individual's personal agency and placing consent at the heart of the practice.

We believe in honoring the complex identities of each member of our community, including pronouns and how people choose to refer to themselves.

We believe trauma-sensitive teaching creates a safer environment for yoga practice.

We believe in practicing asteya—non-stealing—by respecting the roots of the yogic tradition and rejecting cultural appropriation.

We believe in actively uplifting marginalized voices, particularly Black, Indigenous, and People of Color, folks with disabilities, and queer and transgender community members.

We believe that all people—regardless of ability or background—deserve equal access to yoga.

We believe in satya—speaking the truth—and that social justice is yoga in action.

# PART THREE

# YOGA IN PRACTICE

Yoga and its realization are accessible to anyone who commits to its dedicated practice. Perhaps even more important, there is no one, single way to bring about or achieve its transformative insights. Yogic realization is as multifaceted as the participants who practice it. Everyone already belongs to yoga and yoga belongs to everyone.

—MATTHEW SANFORD[1]

# 13 | FINDING YOUR INNER TEACHER

THIS THIRD PART of the book is all about your personal practice. In order to experience the revolutionary aspects of yoga you have to practice—there is no other way. But that practice doesn't have to look the way you may think it does. Yoga is about reaching inside to expose the most tender parts of yourself. First, you expose these parts to yourself, and learn how to care for them. Over time they inform your actions in the world.

Amazingly, your tender heart is your superpower. It's not a weakness, but a strength. If you are sensitive, you can learn how to harness the energy of that special ability and teach the world how to be loving and kind. On the other hand, if you feel out of touch with your feelings, yoga can help to bring them to the surface so you can find a healthy way to process them.

A well-structured yoga practice can offer balance in your life. If you're very busy and have no time, calming practices offer nervous system regulation and relief from the constant stress. If you're feeling tired or worn out, yoga can be invigorating and strengthening.

The chapters in this part offer some general ideas regarding how to bring the fullness of yoga into your life, and chapter 15 outlines a sample practice to offer some ideas for you to explore. This doesn't replace the personal instruction of an experienced teacher, so I hope you'll reach out and find someone to support your journey. Even better, I hope you can find a yoga community to join, in person or virtually, to support your practice and your heart.

> If you're sitting in a chair, maybe sit back a little bit. Your eyes can be open or closed. Wherever you are, you can feel yourself grounded, grounding into the chair or the floor.
>
> On the inhalation, feel length in your spine, lifting. On the exhalation, feel that you're grounding, connecting. Bring your awareness

to the breath. Without changing the breath, see if you can notice the sensations of your breath. Notice what's happening inside your body. Notice the temperature of the air in your nose, the feeling of the movement of air in your throat, expansion in your lungs, movement in your belly.

Be sensitive to the experience of breathing and feel it on an energetic level. Feel how the inhalation fills you with energy and oxygen. The exhalation allows you to release carbon dioxide, letting go. Rest here a moment. Take a deeper inhale and then a slow exhale, slowly opening your eyes if they were closed. Notice how you feel.

## CULTIVATING INTUITION

In the yoga tradition, there is a famous story of a fabled musk deer. This magical animal would spend its life searching for the source of an incredibly appealing fragrance, a musk that it finds overwhelmingly attractive. It literally spends day after day in search of the source of this incredible scent. In snow and wind it climbs over giant mountains just to find the source of the scent, sometimes even plummeting to its death on steep mountain slopes in its desperate search. In a sad and ironic twist, it turns out the musk is being produced by a gland on its own forehead. It was itself the very thing it was desperately looking for. It was the source of its own happiness. In the same way, we spend our lives searching for the source of our happiness in the outer world. Trying to have the right relationships, more money, the right position, or whatever we think might fill the hole in our hearts. We're endlessly searching and searching.

The yoga teachings clearly state that happiness arises from within, and the work of yoga is to be internally focused, rather than externally focused. The idea of finding your inner teacher is the way to cultivate this inner focus. We constantly look to others to be cured, fixed, taught, and made whole. Of course there is a lot to learn about ourselves in relation to others, but eventually we realize, as Alice Walker says, "We are the ones we've been waiting for." We have the wisdom and knowledge within us that we are forever seeking outside.

To cultivate the inner teacher, we explore the relationship between movement and stillness, and between action and inaction, as we become more and more awake to our intuitive knowledge. The experience of increasing our inner awareness is called "interoception," which refers to the perception of sensations inside the body. This inner sensing is a major part of this process and how we hear the voice of that inner teacher.

I always reflect back on the *panchamayakosha* (five bodies) model, which is based on ideas found in the *Taittiriya Upanishad*, an ancient source text that is about 2,000 years old. This model of human embodiment is based on the idea that we have five layers of being, rather than the Western concept of mind and body being two separate things. In the *kosha* model, our essence is expressed in expanding layers moving from subtle to gross. These five layers are: *anandamayakosha* (bliss body), *vijnanamayakosha* (intuitive body), *manomayakosha* (mental body), *pranamayakosha* (energy body), and *annamayakosha* (physical body).

These five bodies, or five layers, are integrated aspects of our human birth. You can't really separate one from the other. But you can influence one layer through the others. This concept of our human embodiment is the basic foundation for the physical practices of yoga. By working on the physical layer we are automatically working with our energy and our mind.

In my practice, the layer that I find most interesting to reflect on is the vijnanamayakosha. This is the body of wisdom, intuition, and inner knowing. At this level of being we connect with the knowledge of life itself: the knowledge of the individual cells in the body that somehow know how to act in unison with billions of others to give us life. The wisdom body is different from the pure consciousness of atman or purusha. The vijnana-mayakosha is embodied awareness, the wisdom of nature and the elements, the body's knowledge.

This is the inner voice that tells us to avoid someone who seems creepy or tells us when to rest and when to act. It's the wisdom of our heart and lungs dancing together to breathe life into our body every moment. It's the wisdom within animals that helps them survive. Recently, a bird known as the bar-tailed godwit was recorded to have flown 7,500 miles in one nonstop marathon migration flight from the Arctic to New Zealand.[1]

It's mind-boggling to consider that the bird flew for eleven days without a break at speeds up to 55 miles per hour. But what I found most incredible is that it knew where to go. The satellite records of its trip showed that it continually made course corrections when the wind blew it off course.

Perhaps there is some simple explanation for this—maybe sensitivity to the earth's magnetic field—but regardless, it's an astounding phenomenon.

It makes me wonder about my body's knowledge. What inner knowing exists locked away in my body? What do my ears, my heart, and my legs know? How do I connect with that knowledge rather than force my body into a top-down practice that I think I'm supposed to do, or that someone else told me to do? How can I cultivate yoga asana organically rather than perform poses?

> Set a timer for five minutes (or longer). Get on your mat, or in a chair if that's where you practice, and begin to allow the body to move without conscious thought about what you're doing. Can you allow your body to move or be still as it wants?

## CREATIVITY IS SPIRITUALITY

Cultural appropriation is when a colonizer takes the practices of an indigenous culture and uses them for its own benefit. There's a fine line between cultural appropriation and what we call cultural appreciation. Appreciation is respecting the culture that the practices come from and giving back in some way. In the case of yoga, it's about not using these practices just for your own benefit, but for the benefit of others. If you approach yoga as service (to yourself as well as others) you can avoid the trap of appropriation by allowing your practice to give you energy to serve.

The fullness of yoga includes lifestyle, asana, meditation, and spirituality. The teachings are diverse and expansive, which is why it's hard to say yoga is just one thing. In fact, we also get stuck when we follow just one lineage of yoga and say it's better than others. As noted earlier, there are many varied lineages that emphasize different aspects of the teachings, such as bhakti yoga, the yoga of devotion; karma yoga, the yoga of selfless action; or jnana yoga, the yoga of wisdom.

Susanna Barkataki, who is considered an expert on cultural appropriation, explains that, "An alternative to cultural appropriation is creativity." Creativity means that we're again connecting to life force, and we're connecting to spirit. Creativity in yoga doesn't mean creating our own style of yoga, rather it means we're reaching into the heart of the practice and connecting to the essence. Creativity means we use the teachings in our own lives to explore and express ourselves. On the other hand, cultural appropriation means that I don't have the ability to find the truth within myself. Instead, I'm just taking someone else's truth and using it for my own personal benefit.

The challenge here is how your practice can be both creative and traditional. It means that if I'm teaching or practicing yoga, and using the word *yoga* instead of *embodied movement*, then I'm connected to an ancient lineage of spiritual seekers who were dedicated to traveling on an inward journey to discover the truth of who they are. The form this journey takes in the world is service, a key element of a traditional practice. It's not that I'm traditional because I only do Ashtanga yoga or Iyengar yoga, but because I'm connected to a tradition of self-reflection and service.

I like to think of yoga as an art more than a science. Art brings in creative expression, which is literally the embodiment of spirituality. Creativity is life force moving through us, and within any art there has to be discipline. Personally, my background is in drawing and painting, and what most people don't realize about art is that it depends on discipline and structure. Generally, you're painting on a rectangular flat canvas, and you're working with a specific limited palette of colors. The discipline of those colors, the two-dimensional surface, and that rectangular space is actually what allows for the creativity to happen. If I paint with every color on every surface, I'll probably just create a huge mess. So creativity needs a structure to work within. Creativity happens with discipline and practice.

In yoga, the discipline is our regular practice. We have particular tools that we use: asana, working with the body; pranayama, working with the breath; and meditation, working with the mind. We also have ethics, philosophy, and service, which allow us to work on our relationships with other people and the world around us. These are the tools of the yoga practitioner that we can use to create a practice that is of use to us, so that we can be useful to the world.

## ACCESSIBLE ASANA

When it comes to asana, we have to remember the goal of yoga is an inner connection. So when we're practicing asana the question becomes, "How is this pose going to support me in connecting with myself?" It could be that it's just fun, and there is a lot of benefit to that. Fun is uplifting and also engages the mind in a powerful way. Making something fun is a great way to keep the mind interested. Or, it could be that a pose creates a challenge. Challenging ourselves can take our full attention. So, in a way, the experience of both fun and challenge can help cultivate a meditative quality.

In the end, asana seems to work even if we don't understand why. It offers us a way of using the body for spiritual practice, which is what makes yoga so special. In most religions and spiritual traditions there's not as much teaching about how to engage the body. Yoga, on the other hand, brilliantly engages us in an embodied spiritual practice. The body and, I would add, the breath are the most powerful tools we have in our practice, and yoga teaches us how to engage them in a productive way. For many people, working with the mind directly such as in meditation or prayer is extremely challenging. The body offers a way inward that circumvents the busy mind. Ironically, asana is what makes yoga accessible and often inaccessible simultaneously.

Patanjali gives us a big hint as to how to practice asana in the few sutras on the topic, even if he's only referring to seated positions. First he explains that, "Asana is a steady, comfortable pose."[2] But the next sutra is astounding. He tells us how to practice: "[Such posture should be attained] by the relaxation of effort and by absorption in the infinite."[3]

Simply being in the present moment, immersed in the body's experience, cultivates yoga. In that way the mind is pulled out of the quicksand of the past, as well as released from the free fall of the future. Our worries, anxieties, and planning all fade for a moment into the awareness of breath, or into the sense of movement in that foot or in that elbow. All an asana has to do is bring our attention to what's happening here and now.

Let's take the example of Eagle Pose, Garudasana. There is so much going on in this pose, which I love. I balance on one foot with the knee of that leg bent. My other leg is wrapped around the standing leg. My arms are crossed tightly and my forearms are wrapped around each other. My back is tall, gaze fixed. Then there's the inner experience of the eagle, perched on a cliff or a tree branch, looking out over a valley. When I practice, I love to open my arms wide on an inhale and on an exhale bring them back together, feeling the opening and closing of wings. Energetically, I exhale and ground downward through the foot of my supporting leg in order to feel the rebounding energy coming back up through my entire body on the inhale. It's a powerful pose that works well to engage my mind.

If you're not comfortable standing you can create this experience sitting in a chair, lying in a bed, or you can simply imagine it in your mind. The benefits of the practice really stem from that subtle shift in energy that happens in the body that captures your attention and draws your mind inward.

One of my favorite ways to practice asana is mentally, without moving the body. Rest in Shavasana (relaxation or Corpse Pose) and imagine yourself in that Eagle Pose (maybe you already have just by reading the description above). Imagine your body in that position. Feel the way your breath moves, and focus your mind. Picturing yourself in the pose will create the experience of yoga because the mind is engaged. It might be even more effective than moving the body!

Visualizing practice exposes the intimate connection between the body and mind. It exposes a basic idea in yoga (connected to the kosha model mentioned above) that there is absolutely no difference between the body and mind. They are just different levels of vibration of the same thing. Recent research in athletes has shown that visualizing practice improves performance because it reduces anxiety. It's intriguing to consider the role of anxiety in our practice and the way that the mind resists being in the present moment.[4]

> Find a resting pose. Then choose one of your favorite asanas. Imagine yourself doing the pose. Inhabit the body while imagining it rather than observing from outside the body. Feel what happens in the body, the sensations, the breath. Then rest and notice how you feel.

## GRAVITY

The effect of gravity is so important to consider when practicing asana. Gravity has much to teach us. The body is always moving in relationship to gravity, and it's this eternal force that we're reckoning with throughout our lives. It's the embrace of Mother Earth holding us tightly to her heart.

Gravity is also the physical experience of time. It can be hard to see time because we're always in the present moment obsessed with remembering the past or fantasizing about the future. But gravity makes time a physical experience. Gravity ages the body in many ways. It's this constant magnetic pull on the body, pulling us back to earth until finally we rejoin her when we die. Gravity can feel like it's crushing me when I'm exhausted. Or in Shavasana, it can feel like a weighted blanket hugging me to the earth.

I sometimes find myself working against gravity in asana and looking at ways to adjust that relationship. My hamstrings are pretty tight, so in a seated forward bend I feel like gravity is pulling me back out of the pose. But if I do a standing forward bend, or legs up the wall, I can create almost the same shape in my body with the energy of gravity guiding me into the pose. The seated forward bend, a practice that often makes me feel anxious, can be transformed into a stable, relaxing experience when working with gravity instead of against it.

Another way to work with gravity in asana is to consider what part of the body is grounding, connecting with the earth, and what part is rising or lifting away. With each exhalation you can feel connected through whatever part of the body is touching the ground. Then as you inhale, you can feel the rest of the body lifting away from the earth.

## INTEROCEPTION: INNER LISTENING

When I train yoga teachers, I often talk about the responsibilities that rest on their shoulders, but it can be very useful to consider the role of the student. As students, we need to have clear boundaries and understand that it's our body, our life, and our practice. The more we can be in touch with our needs, the more effective the experience will be. Rather than giving up our power to the teacher, we engage in a collaborative learning experience: it's a give-and-take. The teacher is making suggestions, and the student is using those suggestions to inform their process. But the authority, or agency, rests in the student to create a practice that is effective, safe, and productive. As M Camellia explains in the sidebar, "My practice has taught me to answer to an internal authority and stand in my innate agency."

With this in mind, I often tell my students, "Listen to me, but don't listen to me." I want them to cultivate inner listening—interoception. This is the awareness of our inner landscape, how we feel inside. It's the ability to feel our own heartbeat, stress level, and emotions. Interoception is one of the most important skills that yoga can give us, as it increases our inner connection. Similarly, proprioception is the ability to know where the body

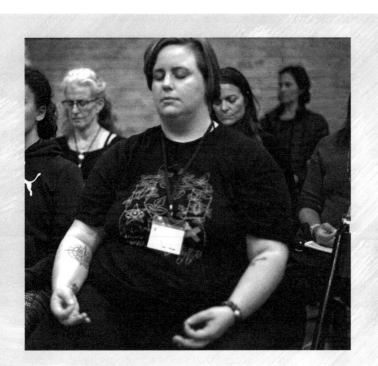

## M CAMELLIA

I've been engaged in social justice work since my teens, but without yoga, my vision was limited. My practice has taught me to answer to an internal authority and stand in my innate agency. By working to reflect my truest, deepest nature instead of mirroring dominant culture, I've begun to understand consent on a deeper level. The divine in me, yoked to our collective divinity, already knows liberation, and it speaks the language of sensation. When I'm acting in alignment with inner wisdom and my unique purpose, I feel it in my body—profound peace and satisfaction, despite any challenges. I call this my divine "yes." At my most discerning, this sensation is my charioteer, driving me to act, explaining my role, and providing direction. To me, this is ishvarapranidhana, a willing surrender of illusory individualism and a commitment to cocreating a just world that elicits a liberated, collective "yes."

is in space. If you extend your arm out at your side, without looking, can you tell whether your hand is level with your shoulder?

Strength and flexibility are not the goals of yoga. Increased self-awareness and peace of mind are what we're seeking. To reach those goals we need to consider the role of asana. Instead of always doing more and pushing further, it's actually agency over our own body, interoception, and proprioception that make for an effective physical yoga practice. And these are the skills that we should focus on as students. In fact, one great practice is to experiment not following a teacher's instructions and see what happens. If you're in a yoga class and you decide to do a different form of a pose, or a different practice altogether, how does that feel for you? Are you willing to stand up for yourself, or are you allowing the teacher's voice to drown out your internal voice? I'm not suggesting that you disrespect the teacher or other students, but can you experiment with finding your own way?

It's also interesting to see how the teacher reacts. Do they get angry if you don't follow every instruction, or do they seem open to sharing power with you? Similarly, if the teacher says, "this practice is so relaxing," and you find it stressful and anxiety producing, what does that tell you? Is your experience wrong, or can you accept that the teacher only has their experience, and they can't know what's happening inside your body?

Pain is another important part of our practice. For some people who have chronic pain, you can't just say, "Stop if you feel pain," since it's constantly present. Instead, someone with chronic pain, and all of us, benefit from increasing our interoceptive ability and becoming more sensitive to that pain, rather than less. In chronic pain, it can be helpful to explore what makes the pain increase and what makes it decrease. Sometimes you won't know right away, and you need to do a practice as best as you can and then notice how you sleep that night and how you feel the next day.

This technique of noticing how you feel the next day is helpful for everyone in finding a practice that is appropriate for your body. The goal isn't to find a practice that doesn't cause any pain, but a practice that over time reduces the experience of pain and offers additional benefit. In the end, a skilled teacher can work with any practitioner to create an accessible practice. Otherwise they're not teaching yoga. As I often say, if it's not accessible, it's not yoga.

# 14 | CARING FOR YOURSELF WITH YOGA

"THEREAFTER ONE IS undisturbed by the dualities."[1] This is how Patan-jali explains the benefit of being established in asana, which always struck me as odd. It's definitely not a benefit you hear many teachers mentioning in class! It's useful to remember that Patanjali's goal was to transcend the world completely—to leave it all behind. These dualities are the ups and downs of life, what make us feel good or bad in any given moment. It's life's roller-coaster ride, which leaves us feeling slightly nauseous and exhausted. Asana helps us realize that you can't have one experience without the other. The dualities are two sides of the same coin.

Up and down, pain and pleasure, hot and cold. These dualities are really one thing: movement, sensation, temperature. As we release our black-and-white thinking we can see the importance of integration as an overarching life goal. Integration is the ability to understand my experience in context, rather than in isolation. *Integration* is another good word for *samadhi*. It's the awareness of the seeming duality of life: nature and spirit, prakriti and purusha. It's the dialectic. The paradox.

I mention this to create context for creating your own yoga practice. Rather than focusing on what you can and can't do physically, try to focus on this idea of integration. Practically speaking, integration represents the glue that holds our life together, connecting all the disparate parts. An effective yoga practice is like connect-the-dots, when you draw the line to connect all the dots and finally an image appears. A practice can provide clarity and perspective, which is a rare gift.

Find a comfortable position and become aware of your breath. No-tice the exhalation. Feel the energy of the exhale moving downward as you connect with gravity and with the earth. Notice your seat and your feet, connecting them to the floor or the chair.

Then notice the inhalation, and feel the energy of the inhale lifting you upward toward the sky. Notice space in the body and between the vertebrae in the spine.

Let the inhale create space and connect you to sky; let the exhale allow you to relax into gravity and connect you to earth.

See if you can find balance in the space between the downward and upward movements. Notice how it feels to allow for opposites to exist at the same time.

## BUILDING A PERSONAL PRACTICE

A yoga practice is made up of two things: formal practice time and the way those practices affect the rest of your life. Formal practice includes the physical practices as well as meditation, scriptural study, prayer, chanting, devotional ceremonies, and more. Most people focus on asana, pranayama (breathing practices), and meditation, which includes guided meditation as well as traditional techniques. In this chapter, I'll discuss creating a formal practice and how you can build a practice that works for you.

The one thing that's essential in a yoga practice is that you begin and end with some form of centering, which is a form of meditation. An opening centering is usually a short meditation, breathing practice, chant, or a body scan. It allows you to bring your full attention to the practice that you're about to do.

A closing centering bookends your practice and allows you to experience the benefits of what you've just done. Personally, at the end of an asana series, I like to end with a short Shavasana (relaxation) or with pranayama and meditation. Or if there's time, all three. I'll offer some suggestions of specific practices in the next chapter, but feel free to incorporate practices that you are already familiar with.

The key is bookending the physical practices with subtle practices. This is important because the subtle practices, and that inner focus, are what makes the practice into yoga. Otherwise, physical practices without inner awareness are really no different than exercise. That's not a bad thing, but it's not really yoga to make shapes with the body without focusing the mind.

Other than an opening and closing centering, I don't think a physical yoga practice has to look any particular way. I find that the opening centering gives me a moment to check in and see what I feel like doing that day. But, I've been doing yoga a long time, and I enjoy changing up my practice and adding additional elements, such as self-massage, dancing, or other kinds of movement. If you're newer to yoga, it may be more effective to create a system that you follow for a little while, so you don't have to think so much. I've created a sample practice in the next chapter that could be a good place to start.

> See if you can make a commitment to yourself to do a formal practice. Try journaling about this idea, and see what arises. Is there resistance? How can you address it?

## A PLACE FOR YOU

So often I hear students complaining about not having enough time in their lives to practice yoga, but I challenge them to think of it in a different way. The formal practice time can become a sanctuary in your life—a place just for you. Personally, I don't think of my practice time as some kind of punishment, rather it's something I look forward to. It's time with myself to check in and see how I feel, and what I need in that moment. It's a respite in my day. I don't think you even have to practice at the same time every day. You can do whatever works for you. I just know that I look forward to my practice time, and by scheduling it at the same time every day, I'm able to work around it.

I find that an afternoon practice works really well with my schedule. I think it's because when my kids were young they got up very early in the morning, and the mornings became a chaotic time with getting them ready for school and all that went with that. I found that late in the afternoon I would generally get tired and need to move my body, which made it conducive to practice. Also, it's when my kids were napping or at an afterschool activity, so it was generally much quieter in our house. I also find that my body is less stiff and less prone to injury in the afternoon than early in the morning, so it feels like a safer time to practice.

The ancient yogis recommended practicing just before dawn, which is a very special time. But most of us are too busy to get up and practice so early in the morning. It is interesting to notice the energy of different times of day. Dusk and dawn both represent that balance in the duality of night and day, sun and moon, which is part of why they are so special.

Finding a special place in your home is similar to finding a special place in your schedule. I realize many people live in tight quarters and don't have the space to roll out a yoga mat. But if possible, see if you can find a corner just for your practice. Over time this space will end up supporting you when you go there, especially if you're feeling down or upset. The energy you invest in your space will feed you later.

## TRUE ALIGNMENT

I'm tired of the judgmental attitude toward using props in yoga. That attitude is part of a competitive approach that feels antithetical to the practice. We're always using props of some kind or another. The floor is a prop, and a yoga mat is a prop. It's completely different to practice on a hard floor versus on grass or in sand on the beach. So often we depend on the resistance of the hard floor without even realizing it.

Actually, the body is itself a prop. If you rest one part of the body on another—as in Eagle Pose with the arms pressing against each other, or in spinal twist when we use the arms and legs to support a twist—you're using the body as a prop. You could even go so far as to say that the body is a prop for the spirit.

Props can be used in so many ways, but mostly they are used to help us avoid injury, which is how I like to think of being in alignment. Being in alignment in asana means that your body is positioned in a way that's not going to injure it. Alignment is not some mystical experience that only advanced yoga practitioners can discover. It's finding the form of the pose that works for your body and makes your practice safe and effective.

As I discussed in the previous chapter, becoming sensitive to your inner teacher is really the best way to avoid injury and reap the most benefit from the practice. It's about becoming more sensitive to what are you feeling, asking yourself, "Would it be better to hold this pose for less time, or for more time? Would it be better to go a little deeper in this pose or back off?" That's how you cultivate that guidance from within.

## CHAIR YOGA

I know it sounds a little strange, but I believe chair yoga is a revolutionary practice. As I've described in detail in this book, the practices of yoga are themselves revolutionary—both inwardly in their potential to change our relationship to ourselves and outwardly in their potential to change the world. Chair yoga offers a way to democratize the practice, making it truly accessible to everyone and touching many more lives with the magic of yoga.

As you can tell, I'm a huge fan of chair yoga. Not only is the practice fun and engaging in a chair, but you can easily access the more subtle practices in a chair. It's not a coincidence that these subtle practices of pranayama and meditation are actually more accessible. Regardless of how your body moves and where you're practicing—whether it's a mat, a chair, or in bed—you can do these practices. They represent the next limbs of ashtanga yoga, taking us into a deeper relationship with ourselves.

When practicing chair yoga, it's usually best to find a solid, strong chair without arms. To make sure you don't fall over, the chair can be against a wall or on a yoga mat to increase traction. Be careful not to lean too far forward in case you might fall out of the chair. You can keep your feet further out in front of you and have your legs wider apart to create a strong base of support.

Also, notice that in chair yoga the body isn't starting from a neutral position like we are in most mat practices. You're starting from a flexed hip and flexed knee position. (That means you're bending forward at the hips and backward at the knees). The flexed hip position tends to cause a slight rounding in the back, decreasing the lumbar curve. That means that you need to be cautious about forward bending, since your spine may already be slightly in flexion, or rounded.

Also, your pelvis is the foundation for the entire upper body when you're seated, and the sit bones are generally a fixed point in any chair yoga pose. That means that the pelvis can't move as freely as it might when you're lying down or standing up. The fixed pelvis is another reason to be sensitive to the lower back and the sacroiliac joint (where the spine connects to the pelvis) in chair yoga.

Try practicing some of the chair yoga poses in the next chapter, paying special attention to the position of the lower back and pelvis. Do you feel how the connection to the chair changes the way that the poses work in the body?

## BED YOGA

As much as I love chair yoga, I'm also passionate about bed yoga. Here is a practice that everyone can do—even people who aren't comfortable sitting up in a chair. But bed yoga isn't just for people with limited mobility. The bed offers a similar surface as the floor, a horizontal plane, so many mat poses can be done in bed without having to transfer to the floor and back up again.

One major issue with practicing in bed is the lack of resistance that the mattress provides. As I mentioned before, a solid floor is a prop that offers support for the body when you're practicing asana. In bed, the softness of the mattress doesn't resist the body, and you may feel like you're sinking down more than you want to. For this reason, it's important to be careful to protect the curves in the spine when practicing in bed. It can help to remove the soft blankets and place a yoga mat on the mattress, creating slightly more resistance.

Bed yoga is a wonderful addition to everyone's practice. You can practice some bed yoga when you wake up in the morning or before you go to bed at night. Moving the body gently, doing some relaxation, gentle breathing, or meditation, can be a great way to wake up or go to sleep. Also, consider how you can find the essence of the practice as you explore creative interpretations and forms—whether it's in bed, in a chair, or on a mat.

Explore some gentle yoga poses in bed. Be especially careful to protect the neck and lower back. Generally, practices done while lying on the back or the sides are most effective.

# 15 | A SAMPLE PRACTICE

HERE IS A SAMPLE practice to support your inner revolution. I'm including mat and chair versions of each of the practices to make them accessible for all levels. In fact, if mat or chair isn't comfortable, most of the mat practices can be done lying in bed. Consider mixing them up or practicing them straight through. I used a few props in this practice that you might want to consider using yourself. This includes one or two chairs, a yoga mat, blankets, a block, and a bolster. If you don't have these props, the practice can be adapted to whatever you have on hand.

As you practice, focus on building awareness of your own body, breath, and mind. Mostly, be kind and sensitive to your own needs. There is a misconception that more is better in yoga, and that's not always the case. Sometimes you need to push yourself to do more, and sometime you just need to rest.

Work on building your interoceptive ability to sense how long to hold each pose and whether to go further or back off. In fact, you don't need to hold the poses at all. Instead try coming into the pose with an inhalation and out of the pose with an exhalation. Repeat a few times and notice how it feels to move rather than to hold a static position. Also, tracking your practice can be very helpful. This can be done in a practice journal or some kind of notebook where you write down what you did and how you're feeling. Over time it can be inspiring to see how you've grown and how yoga has affected your life. Consider journaling about how you're feeling each time you practice, and maybe include some scripture study as part of your routine.

In the following sequence I present the poses in two ways, first using a chair and then using a mat and props where needed. I'm not suggesting you practice both chair and mat versions. Rather, I'm trying to demonstrate that asana can be adapted to you wherever you are right now. Choose a version of the practice that works for you.

Note: If you have any concerns, please consult your health care provider before you begin any physical practices. There are some contraindications to even the most gentle yoga practices. Consider working with a certified yoga teacher or yoga therapist for individual support.

## OPENING CENTERING

### Getting Comfortable

To begin your practice, it's important that you find a comfortable starting position. If you're planning to practice yoga in a chair, then you can use Chair Mountain Pose. If you plan to practice on a mat on the floor you can try sitting in Meditative Pose. Take your time exploring the ways that additional props like blankets and blocks can make you even more comfortable and steady. The focus in all meditation postures is to have the spine long and the rest of the body relaxed.

### Chair Mountain Pose

Sit in a sturdy chair, preferable one that doesn't have arms. Sit slightly forward on the seat of the chair. Or, if you feel like you need support for your back, try sitting all the way toward the back of the seat. Find a position where the spine can be long and the body relaxed.

Notice the relationship of the knees to the hips. Ideally, the knees are about the same height as the hips. If the knees are much lower than the hips, try placing a folded blanket under the feet to raise them up. Or, if the knees are higher than the hips try sitting on a folded blanket to raise the hips.

Have the legs slightly wider than hip-width apart for stability, feet flat on the floor. Also, try having the feet slightly farther out than the knees. This can help keep the body more stable when you're bending forward.

Rest the hands in the lap or on the knees, and check that the body is comfortable for the centering practice.

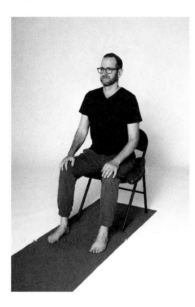

### Meditative Pose

If you're practicing on the mat, sit cross-legged on a bolster, pillow, folded blanket, or blankets. Sit high enough that the lower back feels comfortable.

Place blocks or folded blankets under the knees for extra support and to support the hips. Relax the hands on the lap or on the knees to prepare for the centering practice.

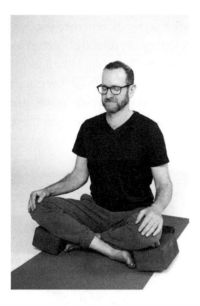

### Centering

You can use a variety of techniques for centering, including chanting, pranayama, silent meditation, guided meditation, intention setting, reading a selection of yoga philosophy, and more.

Chanting is the most traditional form of centering for asana practice. Sometimes the chant is a long invocation of a deity or teacher, and sometimes it's simply OM chanted three times. Experiment with chanting OM slowly, and see if you can feel the sound vibrating in your body. Pay special attention to the *mmm* part of the sound and see if you can feel that vibration all the way up to the top of your head. You can even have your teeth gently touching to increase the vibration.

Also, here's a sample guided meditation you could use:

Have the eyes closed or lower the gaze. Then become aware of what you're feeling through the senses, and see if you can explore your experience without judging it as good or bad.

Notice any sounds in your space. Notice the light coming through the eyes, or what you're seeing if the eyes are open. Notice any sounds. See if you can notice what you're feeling on your skin, maybe the clothing on the body or the temperature of the room. Notice if you smell or taste anything.

Then turn the awareness within and notice the breath. Notice any other sensations inside of the body. Become aware of the mind and any thoughts that you're having. Notice any emotions and see if you can accept all of them without pushing anything away—without judging or criticizing. If there is pain or discomfort, see if you can notice it without turning away.

Don't turn your attention away from what you're experiencing—embrace all of it. Embrace all the sensory input, and embrace all the thoughts or feelings that arise. Embrace the breath, however it is right now, without controlling it. Embrace all aspects of yourself in this moment, not pushing anything away, not denying any part of yourself. You are just being here, completely present with all aspects of yourself. After a few minutes, bring the awareness back to the breath, and then slowly open the eyes if they were closed. Notice how you feel.

## ASANA PRACTICE

### Neck Stretch

Chair Version

To increase mobility in the neck and stretch the neck muscles, you can practice this pendulum-like movement with the head. (Try not to roll the head back.)

Start by inhaling and lengthening the neck, then exhale and lower the chin toward the chest. As you inhale, roll the head to the right side, bringing the right ear toward the right shoulder. On the next exhale, roll the head back down. On the inhale, roll to the left, bringing the left ear toward the left shoulder.

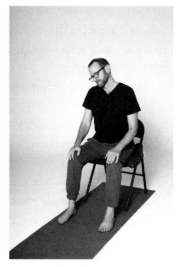

You can continue moving with the breath in this way, or pause at any point where you feel like there is tension. If you find tension, pause, take a breath there and try to release it.

Keep the jaw and shoulders relaxed during the movement. Repeat a few times on each side, and then come back to neutral.

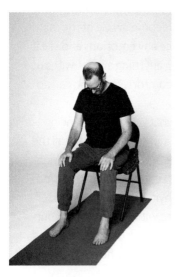

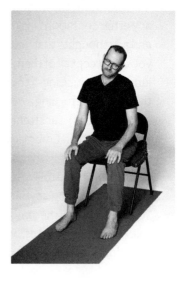

Mat Version

Come to Table Pose for some warm-ups. Place a folded blanket under the knees for extra cushioning. If this is uncomfortable for the wrists you could make fists instead, come down onto your forearms, or place the forearms on the seat of a chair placed in front of you.

To warm up the neck, begin by inhaling and lengthening the neck. As you exhale, slowly lower the head toward the floor. Allow gravity to stretch out the back of the neck.

Keep the jaw relaxed, and slowly begin to roll the head from side to side. You can coordinate the movement with the breath by inhaling to one side and exhaling back down.

Repeat a few times, noticing which positions help to release the most tension.

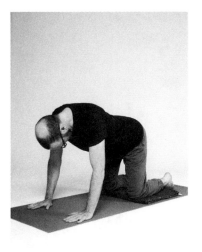
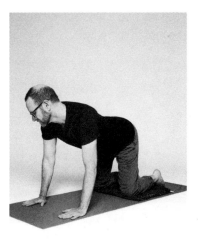

### Hip Circles

Chair Version

To warm up the hip joints, place the left hand on the left knee and begin to make large circles with the knee. Awareness is in the hip joint, which is the deepest ball and socket joint in the body.

Use your hand to support the movement by assisting the leg as it moves. Or gently press the hand into the thigh, creating resistance to the movement. This gentle resistance can be strengthening to the leg muscles. Explore which feels most beneficial right now—assisting or resisting.

Make a few circles in one direction and then go in the other direction an equal number of times. Switch legs and do the same thing with the right leg. Notice the difference between the two sides. After you have done the same amount on both sides, release and notice how the hips feel. If you've recently had a hip replacement, be sure to get advice before working with the hips in this way.

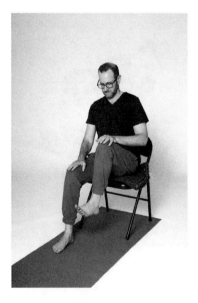
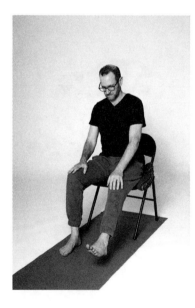

### Mat Version

To do Hip Circles from Table Pose, draw the left knee in toward the chest, and then begin to rotate the knee in a large circle. You can either keep the knee flexed during the entire movement, or extend the leg behind you as you come to that part of the movement. Move the leg slowly, especially as you bring it out to the side so you can notice all the muscles that are coordinating the rotation.

Awareness is in the hip joint. Move the leg slowly in one direction, and then for an equal number of rotations in the opposite direction. Switch legs and do the same movement with the right leg.

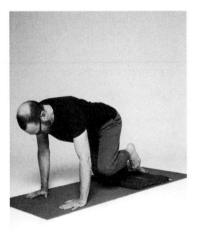 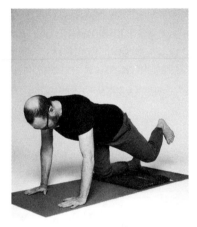

### Foot Stretch

#### Chair Version

Place a block or similar object in front of your chair. Place the toes of the left foot on top of the block toward the edge closest to you. Inhale, and lift the heel up. Exhale, and lower the heel back down toward the floor. Flex and extend the foot with the breath. Practice a few times and then switch sides.

You can do a similar movement by placing the heel on top of the block toward the edge farthest away from you. Inhale, and flex the foot, lifting the toes up. Exhale, and point the foot, lowering the toes toward the floor. Practice very gently, and if you feel like your foot is about to cramp, pause and rest.

A third option is to gently massage the arch of the foot on the edge of the block. To do this, gently press the instep of the foot on the edge of the block. Use a light pressure, and keep lifting the foot off the block repositioning it and pressing it back down. Practice with the other foot.

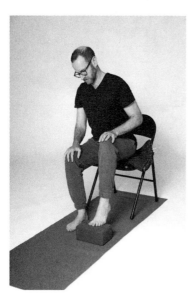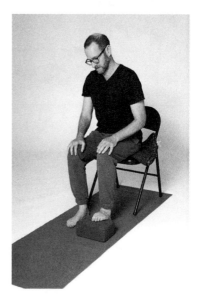

## Mat Version

From Table, extend the left leg out behind you. Inhale, point your toes, and gently rest the top of the foot on the ground. Exhale, flex your foot, lift your toes and press the bottoms of the toes into the floor. Repeat a few times, coordinating the movement with the breath. Then switch to the right leg.

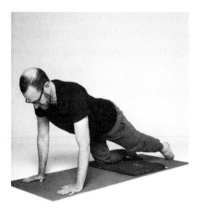 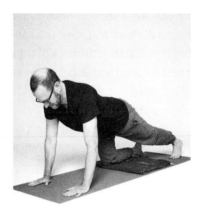

### Cat/Cow

#### Chair Version

Come to Chair Mountain Pose. Place the hands on the knees. To warm up the spine, begin by exhaling and gently rounding the back and lowering the head. Inhale, bring the belly and chest forward and raise the head, looking up slightly.

Repeat these movements again, engaging the arms as well. On the exhale, round the back and see if you can also stretch the hands down past the knees to get a stretch in the back of the shoulders. On the inhale, bring the belly and chest forward and also try to bring the elbows back, opening the front of the chest. Continue this dynamic movement a few times, coordinating the movement and the breath.

Come back to neutral and notice how you feel. Note that spinal flexion, rounding the back and lowering the head, may be contraindicated for osteoporosis and certain kinds of arthritis.

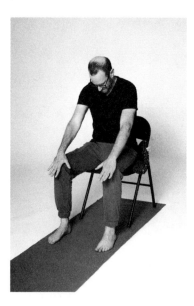 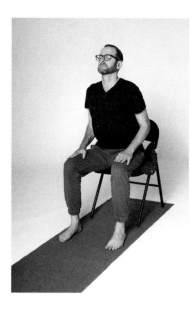

Mat Version

From Table Pose, exhale and tuck the tailbone down. Lift the mid-back up toward the ceiling and lower the head. This is spinal flexion. Inhale, raise the tailbone, lower the belly toward the floor, and lift the head, looking up gently. This is spinal extension.

Continue to coordinate the movement with the breath. Feel that the breath is initiating the movement, and the breath is flowing along the spine as you move. Repeat a few times, slowly, then rest and notice how you feel.

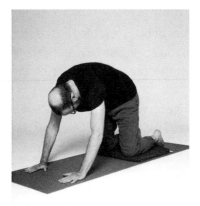 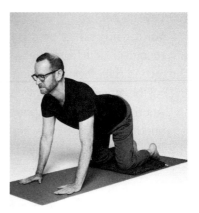

### Child's Pose

Chair Versions

To calm the nervous system, and rest for a moment, you can practice chair Child's Pose. There are a number of different ways to do this practice, so experiment with a few different ones and see which works best for you at this moment.

Place a bolster or folded blanket on your lap. Widen the knees. Hinge forward at the hips and fold the forearms on the bolster. Inhale, lengthen the spine. Exhale, lower the head onto the arms, feeling the gentle pressure at the third-eye center.

You can do a similar practice with a bolster or blanket folded on the seat of a second chair in front of you, facing you. You could also have the back of the second chair facing you, and you can rest the forearms and head on the back of the other chair.

Another way to do this practice is to hinge forward and rest the elbows on your thighs. Interlace your fingers and extend the thumbs. Inhale, lengthen the spine. Exhale, bend the head forward and place the thumbs on the inside corners of the eyebrow ridge.

Feel the gentle pressure massaging you, and try moving the thumbs to different parts of your eyebrows to get an additional massage. Take a few breaths and then release, sitting up and leaning back in the chair to rest.

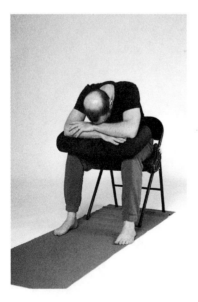
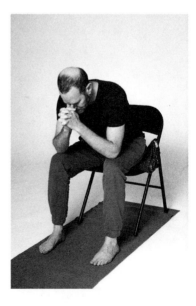

Mat Versions

Come to Table Pose on the mat with a blanket under your shins. Position your-self so your toes are just off the end of the blanket. Widen the knees and sit back toward the heels. If this is uncomfortable on the knees, place a bolster or folded blanket behind the thighs. Inhale, lengthening the spine, exhale, rest the forehead on the floor.

If the forehead doesn't easily reach the floor, place a bolster or other sup-port under the head and chest. If this isn't comfortable, you can place a chair in front of you, with a blanket on the seat. Rest the arms and forehead against the seat of the chair. Or you can practice one of the chair versions above.

Child's Pose, and the gentle pressure on the third-eye area, can help to re-lax the nervous system, but only if you are comfortable and can breathe easily in the pose. This is a gentle inversion, so be aware of any contraindications, such as glaucoma or high blood pressure.

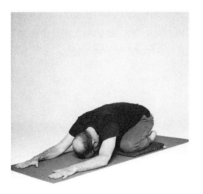 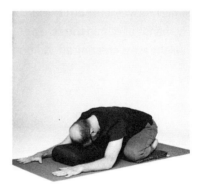

### Cobra Pose

Chair Versions

Cobra can help to strengthen the upper back and neck and can offer relief from "tech neck." From Chair Mountain, place a bolster or folded blanket on your lap. Bring the hands on top of the bolster and hug it gently toward the belly. Hinge forward over the bolster, lowering the head down.

Exhale and feel the gentle pressure on the belly, grounding yourself down into the feet and into the seat of the chair. Inhale, lengthen the spine, and slowly raise up the head and upper chest, rolling the vertebrae up slowly. Bring the awareness to the upper back and the feeling of expansion in the chest. Keep the neck long, and avoid pinching the back of the neck. Take a few breaths here and slowly lower back down. You can repeat again if it felt comfortable.

This variation brings in an abdominal massage, something that can be lost in a chair yoga practice. Another option, without the bolster, is to do a similar movement with the hands on the thighs. Or you can reach back with the hands and hold the side or bottom of the chair, and as you lean forward feel the arms creating an additional stretch to the front of the chest.

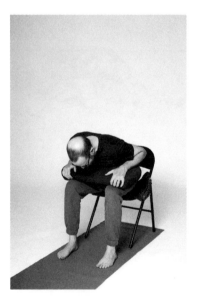 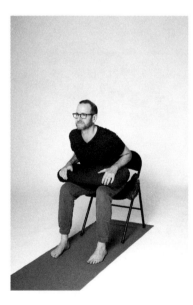

### Mat Version

Fold a blanket so it covers the middle third of the mat (a yoga blanket would be folded in eighths). Place the blanket on the mat so it will be under the front of your pelvis. Lie on your belly, with the blanket under your pelvis. Notice how the blanket helps to lengthen the lower back and reduces the lumbar curve.

Rest with the legs at least hip-width apart, the forehead on the mat, and the hands under the shoulders with the elbows close into the body. Exhale, and press the pelvis into the floor. Inhale, lengthening the spine, engage the back muscles, and slowly raise up the head and upper chest.

Try not to have too much weight on the hands. Don't worry about coming up very far; this is a low cobra designed to access the upper back. Keep the neck long and look forward. Avoid rolling the head back. Take a few breaths here, and then slowly lower back down. If that was comfortable you can repeat again.

Then rest, turn the head to the side, release the arms, and notice how you feel.

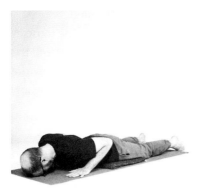
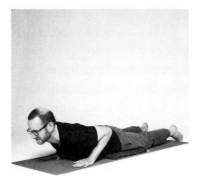

### Tree Pose

Chair Versions

Tree Pose can help with balance, strength, and grounding. You can choose which emphasis you'd like to focus on in your practice. To work with balance, you can experiment with using a soft block or eye pillow on top of your head.

Begin by lengthening the spine. Place the right foot on top of the left thigh. If this is uncomfortable, you can straighten the left leg and lower the right foot down toward the shin. Place the block on your head and hold it with your hands.

Focus the eyes on a spot in front of you. Inhale and lengthen the spine, finding your balance. If you can balance the block, release your hands and bring the palms together at your chest. Take a few breaths here. Release, and practice on the other side, reversing the leg position.

If you want to focus on grounding and strengthening in Tree Pose, try practicing without the prop on your head. You can use a different leg position, such as bringing your right leg out to the side and resting your right heel against the front right leg of the chair, with the toes on the ground.

Lean forward and press the left foot into the floor. Engage the muscles of the left leg, working with isometric strengthening. Inhale, and extend the arms overhead in a Y shape. Exhale and consciously press the left foot into the floor. Take a few breaths here and then release the arms and legs. Notice how you feel. Then practice on the other side.

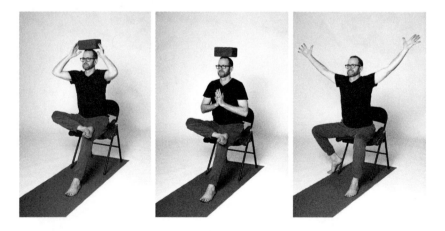

Mat Versions

Come to standing Mountain Pose. This is a neutral position where you are standing on both feet, with the weight balanced, spine long, and the body relaxed. To support your balance, consider standing with your back against a wall or having a chair in front of you, holding the back of the chair for support.

Focus on a spot in front of you with your eyes. Shift the weight to the left leg, softening the knee and engaging the muscles in that leg. Externally rotate the right leg and place the heel of the right foot on the inside of the left ankle with the right toes on the mat.

If you feel balanced, bring your palms together at the chest. Exhale, and feel energy moving down into your left foot, grounding you. Inhale, and feel energy moving up through the top of your head. Take a few breaths in this way, then release the arms and legs and rest.

You can also try practicing Tree Pose with a block under the foot of the raised leg and the arms in a Y position.

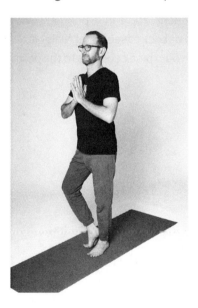 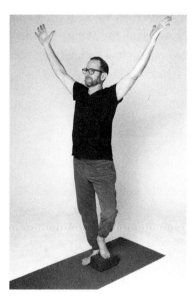

### Triangle Pose

Chair Version

Stretching the side of the body can be calming for the nervous system. Triangle Pose offers this side stretch and can be done in a chair many different ways. One of the most straightforward ways is to begin by widening the legs far apart, with the feet slightly further out than the knees.

From this stable position, rotate the torso to the left. Inhale, and lengthen the spine. Then exhale, and lean to your right, resting the right forearm on the right thigh. The left hand is on the left hip. Focus on the left shoulder and see if you can gently move it back. Keep the neck neutral.

If this is comfortable, you can extend the left arm overhead alongside the left ear. Lengthen from the left hip to the left hand. Take a few breaths here, creating space in the body. Then release and practice on the other side for the same length of time.

In this practice, pay special attention to the lower back, and make sure it feels comfortable throughout the movement. You can experiment with bringing the top of the pelvis gently forward or back to see if that feels better on your sacroiliac joint (the SI joint is where your spine connects to the pelvis in the lower back).

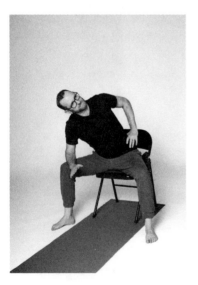
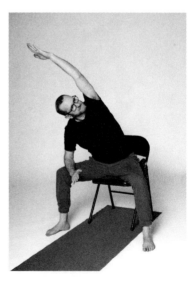

Mat Version

Place a chair, facing you, at one end of your mat. Stand sideways on your mat with the legs wide apart, and the right shin directly in front of the chair. Rotate the right foot out to the side, and as you do so allow the left hip to move forward a little. For more stability, you can move your right foot closer to the edge of the mat behind you.

Extend the arms out at shoulder height. Take a breath here. Inhale, feeling length through the spine. Then as you exhale, reach out with the right hand and begin to lower down to the right. Place the right hand on the seat of the chair and the left hand on your left hip.

Notice how your lower back feels, and if it's uncomfortable, try bringing your left hip slightly forward or back. Take another breath, lengthening the spine, neck neutral, creating space on the left side of the body. Try to rotate the left shoulder back, expanding the chest.

If this is comfortable, on the next inhale, stretch the left arm overhead, alongside the left ear. Take a few breaths here, and then come up slowly and release the arms and bring the legs back together. Turn to face the other side of your mat and practice on the other side of your body.

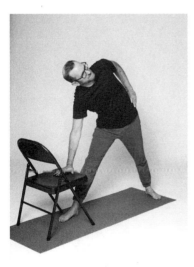
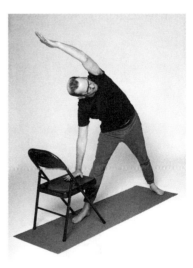

### Twist

#### Chair Versions

Twisting the spine can help to keep the spine flexible and retain a healthy range of motion in the spinal joints. It can also stretch the hips and shoulders, but I suggest beginning with a twist that relies on the back muscles, rather than the strength of the arms.

One example of this is a chair Twist done by crossing the left leg over the right thigh or ankle. Bring the palms together at the chest. Inhale, lengthen the spine, and on the exhalation begin twisting to the left side. You may not go as far as you'd expect without using the arms to assist you, but this practice helps to engage and strengthen the muscles along the spine. Take a few breaths here and then release. Practice for the same amount of time on the other side.

Another option is to use the arms for support. In this practice, cross the legs at the thighs or ankles. Place the right hand on the left knee. Inhale, lengthen the spine. Exhale, twist to the left and place the left hand on the back of the chair, or on the back of the seat of the chair behind the hips. Keep the chest expanded and the shoulders relaxed. Take a few breaths here and then release.

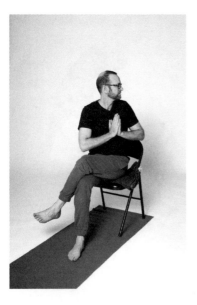 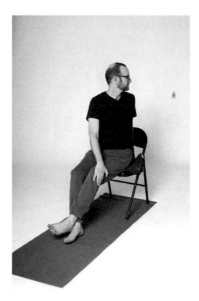

### Mat Versions

Similar to the chair Twist, you can practice a seated Twist on the mat that emphasizes engagement of the back muscles. For this practice, try sitting in a comfortable cross-legged position with the palms together at the chest. Inhale, lengthen the spine, and as you exhale, twist to the left. Bring the left shoulder back and look gently over the left shoulder. Take a few breaths here, and then practice on the other side.

This could also be done dynamically, which means moving with the breath. Begin sitting facing forward. Inhale, lengthen the spine. Exhale, twist to the left. Inhale, come back to center. Exhale, twist to the right. Continue twisting to either side, coordinating the movement and the breath.

You can also practice with the help of the hands. Sitting cross-legged, facing forward, place the right hand on the left knee. Bring the left hand to the left hip, or to the floor behind you. Inhale, lengthen the spine, and exhale, twist to the left. Stay here for a few breaths, focusing the twist on the middle and upper back. Try not to force the twist with the arms.

You can also experiment with the legs extended in a more traditional half spinal twist. Avoid twisting in the lower back. In fact, to protect the SI joint, you could try moving the hip of the side your twisting to slightly back.

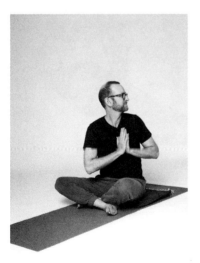 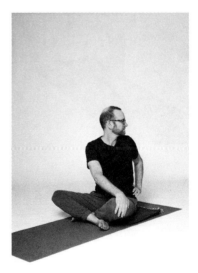

### Pigeon Pose

Chair Version

From chair Mountain Pose, take the left foot and cross it on the top of the right thigh. If this is uncomfortable, you can straighten the right leg and place the left foot lower down along the right leg.

Hold the left knee with the left hand and left foot with the right hand. Flex the left foot to protect the knee. Inhale, lengthen the spine. Exhale, gently bend forward over the legs until you feel a stretch in the left hip.

Take a few breaths here, exploring the sensation in the hip and being careful not to overstretch. Inhale and sit back up, releasing the leg back down. Practice on the other side.

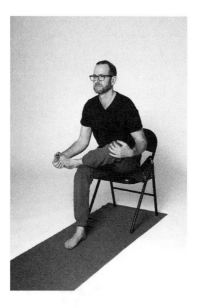 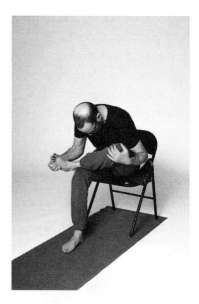

Mat Versions

Start in Table Pose, and place a bolster across the mat just in front of the knees. Lift the right leg up and over the bolster, placing it down on the mat. Move the right foot toward the left so the bolster is underneath the hips. Move the right leg around to find a comfortable position, or if this isn't comfortable, try practicing the next version on your back or chair Pigeon.

Inhale and lengthen the spine, being careful not to overly arch the back. Exhale, and gently lean forward, bringing the forehead to the floor or to a block or other prop. The arms can rest down onto the floor to help relax the shoulders.

Pay attention to the right hip and knee, and make sure you're not straining. Take a few breaths here, and then slowly rise back up. Bring the right leg back, coming into Table again. Repeat on the other side, noticing the difference between the two sides.

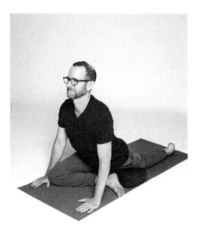
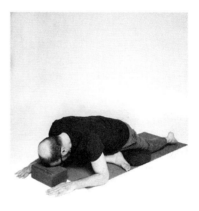

For a gentler hip stretch, you can practice a variation of Pigeon Pose on your back. For this practice, begin lying in Shavasana, Relaxation Pose. Bend both knees with the feet on the mat. Cross the left foot onto the front of the right thigh. Flex the left foot to protect the left knee.

If comfortable, reach down and take hold of the right thigh with both hands. Bring the legs toward the chest, increasing the stretch without straining. Keep the shoulders relaxed and the head down. You could place a folded blanket under the head if that's more comfortable. Stay here for a few breaths and then release slowly. Practice on the other side for the same amount of time.

Another variation is to not hold the leg with the hand. Instead, bend both knees with the feet on the mat. Place a block under the right foot. Place the left foot on the front of the right thigh, keeping the foot flexed. In this version, see if you can find a position that you can hold for slightly longer, giving the hip muscles time to relax.

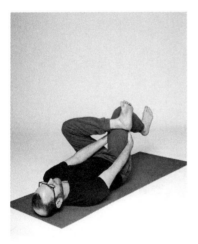
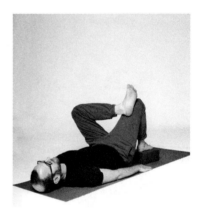

## RELAXATION

### Relaxation Pose

Chair Versions

The Relaxation Pose in yoga is Shavasana, which means "corpse pose." For chair relaxation, the goal is to find a position that is both comfortable and steady. It can be challenging to find a position in a chair that allows the body to completely let go. So, it's worth exploring a few different options.

If you're practicing at home, you may want to lie in bed, or on a couch, to allow the body to be completely supported. In a chair, focus on supporting the spine and the neck. You can move your chair in front of a wall, and rest the head back against a wall. Or use pillows or folded blankets behind the back for support.

You can also raise the legs on a bolster or second chair. Try placing a bolster or folded blanket on the lap. Having a prop on the lap is surprisingly effective for supporting relaxation. Similarly, it can be very powerful to cover yourself with a blanket, even if you're not cold. The weight of the blanket, or bolster, can help the body relax.

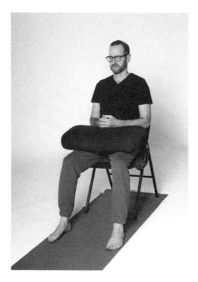
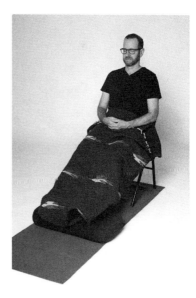

### Mat Versions

As I've mentioned before, relaxation depends on safety, quiet, darkness, and a comfortable temperature. Take some time to prepare by finding a space that will be conducive to relaxation. If you're practicing on the floor, gather the props you'll need and lie down on your back. Generally, most people like to have support under the neck and knees. Experiment with different heights of support to find what's most effective for you.

One way to use a flat bolster is to place it under the knees on its long thin side. Once you're lying back, see if you can allow the top of the bolster to fall toward your feet. As it does so, the bolster will gently pull on the backs of the knees, offering a slight traction to the lower back.

You might want to cover yourself with a blanket and use an eye pillow to block out the light. Sometimes a bolster or folded blanket over the belly can be comforting. Also, spend some time working with the position of the arms and hands—even propping the backs of the wrists with a small pillow or support can help to release the shoulders slightly.

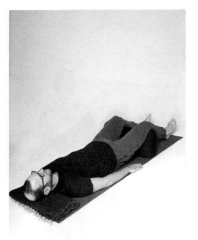
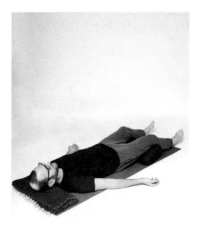

### Guided Relaxation

Once the body is in a comfortable position, spend some time simply resting quietly or in a guided relaxation or *yoga nidra* practice. Yoga nidra is a type of meditation where you are guided through the different bodies, the koshas; other approaches use a variety of relaxation techniques. You can find recorded yoga nidra or guided relaxations online, or you can guide yourself by using a recording.

One effective technique is to find the script for a relaxation that you like, or write your own. Then record yourself reading through the script slowly and play it back. There is something very powerful about hearing your own voice instructing you to let go.

There are a few general guidelines you could use if you're creating your own guided relaxation. These don't need to be intricate. It can simply be a minute of rest or fifteen minutes of guided instruction.

- Body scan: Bring awareness to different parts of the body. Generally, from outer to inner, from the feet up. Go slowly.
- From gross to subtle: Move from the physical body to the breath (energy body), to the mind, to the witness, and finally to the peace within.
- Silence: Spend the last part of the relaxation in silence. This could be just for a moment or a few minutes.
- Use positive, general images that don't stimulate the mind, but allow it to relax.
- Come out slowly.

## PRANAYAMA

Pranayama, breathing practices, give us access to the subtle energy, or prana, in the body. These are powerful practices that can affect the nervous system and the mind. Be very gentle with yourself, and if you feel uncomfortable at any time just stop and relax the breath.

Additionally, breathing practices can release emotion or stored memories. So for people who have had trauma or have anxiety, these practices should be approached very carefully. Just as they offer tremendous healing potential, they can also be triggering.

The best thing is to start slowly and simply. In fact, the basic pranayama is deep breathing. This is actually an introductory practice before you get into formal pranayama, but it offers tremendous benefit. The idea is to become more sensitive to your breath, and if comfortable, to expand it slightly.

The power of pranayama comes through subtlety, not through big, aggressive changes. Sometimes it may feel like nothing is happening, but as long as you're aware of the breath or energy, then something is happening.

### Deep Breathing

Sit in a comfortable position, either in the chair or on the mat, and place one hand on your belly and one on your chest. First notice how the breath is moving. Then deepen the breath just slightly. Begin with an exhalation, and feel the belly moving in toward the spine. As you inhale, feel the belly moving forward, away from the spine. Do this a few times. Then, on an inhale, feel the belly move forward and the breath expand up into the chest, expanding the lungs. Exhale from the chest and then feel the belly moving in.

Continue in this way for a few more breaths. Feel the belly and chest expand on the inhale. You can even feel the collarbones rise. On the exhale, feel the chest and belly contract. Then relax the breath and release the hands. Spend a moment noticing how you feel.

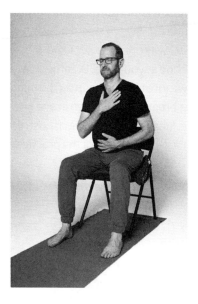
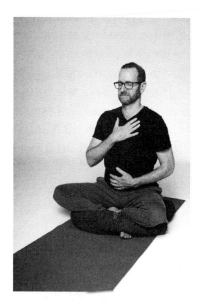

### Alternate Nostril Breathing

Practicing with the Mind

Alternate nostril breathing, *nadi shuddhi* or *nadi shodhana*, is a powerful practice for calming the nervous system and relaxing the mind. This is one of the safest pranayama practices, and also one of the most effective.

This practice can be done with or without the hands closing the nostrils. First, I'll describe it without touching the nose, just using the mind to control the breath. This version of the practice depends on deep concentration so you can visualize the breath moving in and out of each nostril. This focused attention is one of the reasons this form of the practice is so effective.

Sit in a comfortable position with the hands face up on the lap in gentle fists. Using the power of your mind, imagine the breath leaving from the right nostril. As you exhale, slowly open the right hand. Then inhale through the right nostril and slowly close your hand into a gentle fist. Switch sides and imagine the breath leaving from the left nostril as you slowly open the left hand. Inhale from the left nostril and slowly close the left hand as you do so. Breathe slowly.

Continue to practice in this way for a few more rounds, keeping the mind completely focused on the movement of the breath out and then in one nostril at a time. Remember the pattern is exhale, inhale, and then switch nostrils. After you've finished, sit for a moment and notice the effects of the practice.

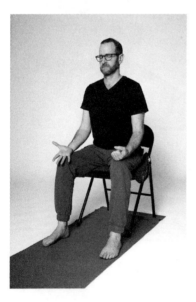 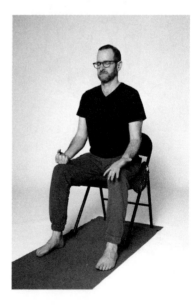

Practicing with the Hands

Traditionally, alternate nostril breathing is done by using the fingers to close one nostril at a time. The traditional hand position is called Vishnu mudra, named for the deity Vishnu, whose name means "all-pervading." Making a gentle fist with the right hand, extend the pinky, ring finger, and thumb. Bring the hand to the face and close the right nostril with the thumb, exhaling from the left side. Inhale from the left nostril, then close it with the ring finger, release the thumb and exhale from the right nostril. Go slowly.

Continue with this same pattern for a few minutes. The focus is on calm, slow breathing. If you feel short of breath or uncomfortable in any way, release the hand and return the breath to normal.

After a few minutes, release the hand and relax the breath. Notice how you're feeling. If the Vishnu mudra isn't comfortable, you can use the index finger and the thumb instead. Similarly, if using the right hand isn't comfortable for you, try using the left hand.

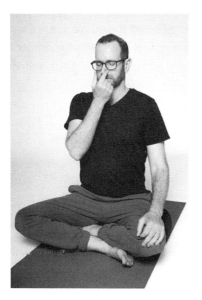 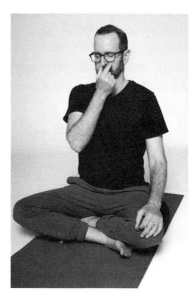

### Ocean Breathing

One additional practice to begin with is *ujjayi*, which is also referred to as ocean breathing. This practice is the best way to learn how to slow the breath, which in turn, slows the mind and calms the nervous system. These are the major benefits of pranayama and why these practices are so effective at calming the mind.

Ocean breathing is done by closing the glottis slightly, making a very light wheezing sound in the throat. Sometimes this is called Darth Vader breathing, but that is really too loud a sound. Ujjayi works best when it's so subtle that you can barely hear it. It's more a matter of awareness in the throat, giving us a little control over the rate of breathing. It's an energetic experience more than a forceful effort.

It's easiest to begin by using ujjayi on the exhalation. To practice, inhale normally, and then on the exhale try to make a slight wheezing sound. See if this sound allows you to lengthen the exhale. Make it as long as you comfortably can, and notice how the slow exhale quickly calms the nervous system.

Do a few rounds of ujjayi focusing on lengthening the exhale. Eventually, this practice can be combined with alternate nostril breathing. Experiment with lengthening the breath, making sure that you're not straining at any time. Always pause after you practice to notice how you're feeling.

## MEDITATION

### Meditation Poses

Chair Versions

Here are a few different seated positions you can use for meditation, although it really doesn't matter what position you are in. What's most important is that the body is comfortable and relaxed and not distracting you. You can also use one of the positions discussed earlier under Getting Comfortable.

You can sit in chair Mountain with the hands resting in the lap, or you can try using *chin* mudra. (The name *chin* means consciousness, not the chin on your face.) In this hand position, have the palms facing up and touch the index finger to the thumb. Mudras are powerful gestures that allow prana, or energy, to flow in particular patterns in the body.

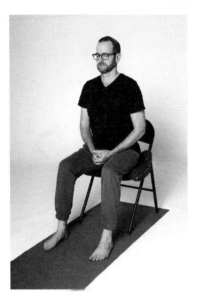 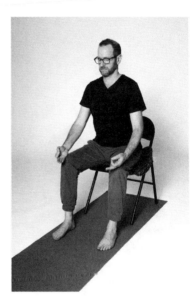

### Mat Versions

On the mat, you can try a variety of positions for seated meditation. Again, the most important thing is that your body is comfortable and not distracting you. You can sit in a cross-legged position and use support under the knees, such as blocks or folded blankets.

One of my favorite props for sitting on the floor is a rolled blanket wrapped over the feet and under the knees. This helps to support the hips and cushion the feet and ankles as well. You can see a picture of this under Closing Centering.

Another traditional posture, Siddhasana, involves bringing one foot in front of the other, rather than tucking them under the thighs. You can also use a kneeling position, supported by props, or lean back against a wall. Spend some time finding a position that is comfortable for you, so that you can relax into your meditation.

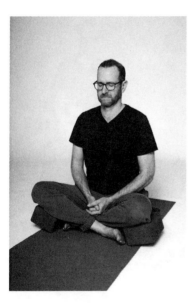
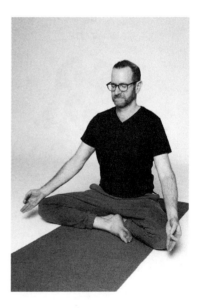

### Meditation Techniques

As I've discussed earlier, meditation is an essential part of yoga practice. Unfortunately, it's often not included in public yoga classes, and many people have a fear of meditation because they think it means they need to get their mind to be quiet. Controlling the mind may be one of the goals of meditation, but it's not the way in.

The way we start to meditate is by becoming friendly with the mind and accepting it for what it is. Otherwise, you're setting yourself up for failure and frustration. Meditation is not a time to judge yourself or practice self-sabotage. It's a time to sit with yourself, just like you would sit with someone you love and enjoy their presence.

There are so many techniques to try, but in the end it all comes back to that relationship with yourself. Meditation is time to listen to the voice of your heart: if you can open yourself to listening, rather than talking, then you are meditating.

You can try focusing the mind on the breath, or a mantra like OM SHANTI, which means "peace." Or you can stare at a flower or an uplifting picture. But, what's most important is that you spend a moment with yourself being absolutely present. This is a chance to enjoy the benefit of all the work you've just done with your asana and pranayama practice. That preparation can make meditation much more comfortable and effective—even if it's only for a brief moment of deep listening.

Take a moment to sit with yourself and listen. Begin with noticing the body and making sure it's comfortable. Then take a deep breath in, pause for a moment, and as you exhale see if you can release a sense of gripping or tightness in the body, and in the mind. Take a few more breaths in this way if it feels helpful. As the tension releases, feel open to exploring your inner world. This means allowing the mind to stop talking for a moment so there is space to listen to any subtle messages or feelings. Simply notice whatever you discover without judgment. There's no goal nor good or bad way to be present with yourself. When the mind starts talking, see if you can ask it to listen instead. Spend just a few minutes here. Take another deep breath in and long slow exhale. Slowly come out of your meditation and notice how you feel.

## CLOSING CENTERING

It's important to end your practice as you began, with centering. This means you end with a moment of reflection, a short meditation, or a chant. This can be one of the practices I've just discussed or a combination of practices. A closing centering may be different than an opening centering in one important way: it usually includes a dedication. This means we dedicate the results of our practice to something other than our own ego-mind.

This dedication or offering could be a prayer for someone we love or for the entire universe. By offering the practice in this way, we can turn our practice itself into a form of service to others. A few forms of closing centering could be:

- Bring the palms together in Anjali mudra and bow to the teacher within
- Chant three OMS or OM SHANTI, SHANTI, SHANTI. *Shanti* means "peace."
- Chant a sacred prayer like the Asatoma mantra (37) or another prayer that is meaningful to you. One of the most sacred mantras is the Om Tryambakam mantra, from the Rig Veda, which is often associated with healing and purification. It's a prayer to Lord Shiva to release us from death.

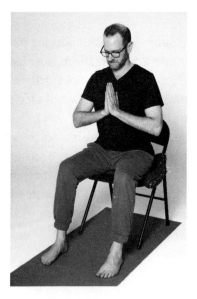 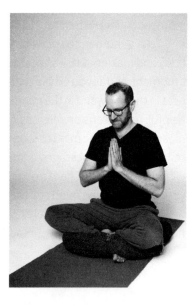

Om tryambakam yajaamahe
sugandhim pushti vardhanam
urvaarukamiva bandhanaan
mrityor moksheeya mamritaat
(repeat 3 times)

Om shanti, shanti, shanti

We worship the All-seeing One
Fragrant, you nourish bounteously.
From the fear of death may you cut us free
To realize immortality.

Om peace, peace, peace[1]

# SUMMARY OF PART THREE

THE PARADOX OF YOGA is that it is an embodied spirituality. We use the body and the mind to transcend their own limitations. We do lots of poses, breathing practices, and meditation to create a foundation for cultivating real change in our lives. Sometimes we get lost in the physical practices and forget that they have a spiritual purpose. It's okay to forget, but it makes the practices more effective if we can simply remember their underlying goal.

This isn't about rejecting the body and mind, but loving them even more. By embracing our body and mind, we can build a stronger relationship with ourselves. After all, the body and mind are the vehicle for our spirit, and should be treated as such—not adulated nor denigrated, but cared for with love and compassion. A balanced yoga practice makes the body and mind more flexible, stronger, and resilient to the challenges of life, and it makes us ready to serve our highest calling.

My interest is in showing you the connections between your personal practice and the way you perceive yourself and the world around you. If you perceive yourself as a completely separate entity, only concerned about your own safety and happiness, then you're not practicing yoga. You can do all the sun salutations that you want, but it won't change that.

Instead, you need to dive a little bit deeper—into the teachings, and into yourself. You're not only connected to everyone else; you're connected to the whole universe. In fact, according to the *Chandogya Upanishad*, which is over 2,500 years old, you have the entire universe inside of you:

> The little space within the heart is as great as this vast universe. The heavens and the earth are there, and the sun, and the moon, and the stars; fire and lightning and winds are there; and all that now is and all that is not: for the whole universe is in Him and He dwells within our heart.[1]

I hope the awareness of that little space within your heart increases your capacity for self-love and for service. I also hope you'll allow yoga to work on you. The way yoga works depends on your life experience and what you're bringing to the practice. If you have been oppressed, or have trauma, yoga can become a sanctuary of healing to give you back some of the agency and power you may feel that you have lost. Of course, this is dependent on your ability to create a practice that empowers you, rather than one that continues to make you feel less than, or traumatized.

If you have power and privilege, then yoga can help open your heart and mind to other people's experiences. I heard a great analogy the other day: If the Supreme Court has never decided a case that personally affects your basic human rights, then you have a lot of privilege. In that case, you have an even greater responsibility to share power with others—that is your yoga. The fact is, most of us have complex identities that straddle both privilege and oppression. We all need a practice that is personally healing and allows us to have compassion for others.

The three parts of this book reflect the way that yoga can work on us individually and contribute to our communal awakening. It starts with a personal practice grounded in the teachings—a practice that will support your work in the world. This practice will literally focus your mind, as well as your energy (prana), toward fulfilling your dharma. That means you will be more effective at whatever work you do in the world.

The secret of yoga is that true happiness only comes if you focus that energy on service. Through service—by thinking of the welfare of others—you are literally transforming love into action. By doing so, you get to bask in that love yourself. The more you give the more you get is the fundamental principle of these teachings.

With these tools, yoga can transform our lives, and in doing so, it can change the world. Millions of people practice yoga every day, but how many practice the spiritual teachings of yoga? If we all took these essential teachings to heart, we could create a world filled with compassion and love for all.

# RESOURCES

## THE YOGA SUTRAS OF PATANJALI
*\*I've added an asterisk next to titles that are most useful for beginners.*

\*Adele, Deborah. *The Yamas & Niyamas: Exploring Yoga's Ethical Practice.* Duluth, MN: One-Word Bound Books, 2009.

Bachman, Nicolai. *The Path of the Yoga Sutras: A Practical Guide to the Core of Yoga.* Boulder, CO: Sounds True, 2011.

\*Bryant, Edwin F. *The Yoga Sutras of Patanjali: A New Edition, Translation, and Commentary.* New York: North Point Press, 2009.

\*Carrera, Reverend Jaganath. *Inside the Yoga Sutras.* Yogaville, VA: Integral Yoga Publications, 2006.

\*Devi, Nischala Joy. *The Secret Power of Yoga.* New York: Three Rivers Press, 2007.

Feuerstein, Georg. *The Yoga Sutra of Patanjali: A New Translation and Commentary.* Rochester, VT: Inner Traditions International, 1989.

Finger, Alan. *Tantra of the Yoga Sutras: Essential Wisdom for Living with Awareness and Grace.* Boulder, CO: Shambhala Publications, 2018.

Hariharananda Aranya, Swami. *Yoga Philosophy of Patanjali.* Albany: State University of New York Press, 1983.

Hartranft, Chip. *The Yoga-Sutra of Patanjali: A New Translation and Commentary.* Boston, MA: Shambhala Publications, 2003.

Iyengar, B. K. S. *Light on the Yoga Sutras of Patanjali.* London: Thorsons, 2002.

Miller, Barbara Stoler. *Yoga Discipline of Freedom: The Yoga Sutra Attributed to Patanjali.* New York: Bantam Books, 1998.

Prabhavananda, Swami, and Christopher Isherwood. *How to Know God: The Yoga Aphorisms of Patanjali.* Hollywood, CA: Vedanta Society, 1981.

\*Ranganathan, Shyam. *Patanjali's Yoga Sutra.* Haryana, India: Penguin Books, 2008.

Ravindra, Ravi. *The Wisdom of Patanjali's Yoga Sutras: A New Translation and Guide*. Sandpoint, ID: Morning Light Press, 2009.

Remski, Matthew. *Threads of Yoga: A Remix of Patanjali's Sutras with Commentary and Reverie*. Matthew Remski, self-published, 2012.

Roy, Ranju, and David Charlton. *Embodying The Yoga Sutra: Support, Direction, Space*. Newburyport, MA: Weiser Books, 2019.

*Satchidananda, Swami. *The Yoga Sutras of Patanjali*. Yogaville, VA: Integral Yoga Publications, 2003.

Stiles, Mukunda. *Yoga Sutras of Patanjali*. Boston, MA: Red Wheel/Weiser Books, 2001.

Tigunait, Pandit Rajmani, PhD. *The Practice of the Yoga Sutra: Sadhana Pada*. Honesdale, PA: Himalayan Institute, 1998.

———. *The Secret of the Yoga Sutra: Samadhi Pada*. Honesdale, PA: Himalayan Institute, 1998.

Vivekananda, Swami. *Raja Yoga*. New York: Ramakrishna-Vivekananda Center, 1982.

## THE BHAGAVAD GITA

Cox, Ted L. *Warrior Self: Unlocking the Promise of the Bhagavad Gita*. Oklahoma City: Spirit House Yoga Publishing, 2014.

*Easwaran, Eknath, *The Bhagavad Gita*. Tomales, CA: Nilgiri Press, 2007.

Gandhi, Mohandas K. *The Bhagavad Gita According to Gandhi*. Berkeley, CA: Berkeley Hills Books, 2000.

Mascaro, Juan. *The Bhagavad Gita*. London: Penguin Books, 1962.

Mitchell, Stephen. *Bhagavad Gita: A New Translation*. New York: Three Rivers Press, 2000.

Prabhavananda, Swami, and Christopher Isherwood. *Bhagavad Gita*. Bloomington, IN: Barnes & Noble Books, 1995.

Ravindra, Ravi. *The Bhagavad Gita: A Guide to Navigating the Battle of Life*. Boulder, CO: Shambhala Publications, 2017.

*Satchidananda, Swami. *The Living Gita: The Complete Bhagavad Gita*. New York: Henry Holt & Company, 1990.

Schweig, Graham M. *Bhagavad Gita: The Beloved Lord's Secret Love Song*. New York: Harper Collins, 2007.

Stoler Miller, Barbara. *The Bhagavad-Gita: Krishna's Council in Time of War*. New York: Bantam Books, 2004.

Viljoen, Edward. *The Bhagavad Gita: The Song of God Retold in Simplified English*. New York: St. Martin's Press, 2019.

## ADDITIONAL BOOKS

Arbinger Institute, The. *The Anatomy of Peace: Resolving the Heart of Conflict*. Oakland, CA: Berrett-Koehler Publishers, Inc. 2020.

Arora, Indu. *Yoga: Ancient Heritage, Tomorrow's Vision*. Minneapolis, MN: YogSadhna Inc. 2019.

Ballard, Jacoby. *A Queer Dharma: Your Liberation Bound with Mine*. Berkeley, CA: North Atlantic Books, 2021.

Barkan, Ady, *Eyes to the Wind: A Memoir of Love and Death, Hope and Resistance*. New York: Atria Books, 2019.

Barkataki, Susanna. *Embrace Yoga's Roots: Courageous Ways to Deepen Your Yoga Practice*. Orlando, FL: Ignite Yoga and Wellness Institute, 2020.

Bell, Baxter, and Nina Zolotow. *Yoga for Healthy Aging: A Guide to Lifelong Well-Being*. Boulder, CO: Shambhala Publications, 2017.

Bondy, Dianne. *Yoga for Everyone: 50 Poses for Every Type of Body*. Indianapolis, IN: DK Books, 2019.

Bondy, Dianne, and Kat Heagberg. *Yoga Where You Are: Customize Your Practice for Your Body and Your Life*. Boulder, CO: Shambhala Publications, 2020.

brown, adrienne maree. *Emergent Strategy: Shaping Change, Changing Worlds*. Chico, CA: AK Press, 2017.

Clampett, Cheri, and Biff Mihoefer. *The Therapeutic Yoga Kit: Sixteen Postures for Self-Healing through Quiet Yin Awareness*. Rochester, VT: Healing Arts Press, 2009.

Corn, Seane. *Revolution of the Soul: Awaken to Love through Raw Truth, Radical Healing, and Conscious Action*. Boulder, CO: Sounds True, 2019.

Dark, Kimberly. *Damaged Like Me: Essays on Love, Harm, and Transformation*. Stirling, UK: AK Press, 2021.

Desikachar, T. K. V. *The Heart of Yoga: Developing a Personal Practice*. Rochester, VT: Inner Traditions International, 1995.

Emerson, David, and Elizabeth Hopper, PhD. *Overcoming Trauma through Yoga: Reclaiming Your Body*. Berkeley, CA: North Atlantic Books, 2011.

Farhi, Donna, *Teaching Yoga*. Berkeley, CA: Rodmell Press, 2006.

Frankl, Viktor E. *Man's Search for Meaning: An Introduction to Logotherapy*. New York: Simon & Shuster, 1984.

Freire, Paulo. *Pedagogy of the Oppressed.* London: Penguin Classics, 1993.

Gandhi, Arun, *The Gift of Anger: And Other Lessons from My Grandfather Mahatma Gandhi.* New York: Jeter Publishing. 2017.

Hanh, Thich Nhat. *Being Peace.* Berkeley, CA: Parallax Press, 1987.

Johnson, Michelle Cassandra. *Finding Refuge: Heart Work for Healing Collective Grief.* Boulder, Shambhala Publications, 2021.

———. *Skill in Action: Radicalizing Your Yoga Practice to Create a Just World.* Portland, OR: Radical Transformation Media, 2017.

Klein, Melanie. *Yoga Rising: 30 Empowering Stories from Yoga Renegades for Every Body.* Woodbury, MN: Llewellyn Publications, 2018.

Krishnamurthi J. *Think on These Things.* New York: Harper & Row 1989.

Ladinsky, Daniel. *The Gift: Poems by Hafiz, the Great Sufi Master.* New York: Penguin Group, 1999.

Landreman, Lisa M. *The Art of Effective Facilitation: Reflections from Social Justice Educators.* Sterling, VA: Stylus Publishing, 2013.

Mallinson, James, and Mark Singleton. *Roots of Yoga.* London: Penguin Classics, 2017.

Mascaro, Juan. *The Upanishads.* London: Penguin Books, 1965.

Menakem, Resmaa. *My Grandmother's Hands: Racialized Trauma and the Pathway to Mending Our Hearts and Bodies.* Las Vegas, NV: Central Recovery Press, 2017.

Mohan, A. G., and Dr. Ganesh Mohan. *Hatha Yoga Pradipika.* Svastha Yoga, 2017.

Nietzsche, Friedrich. *Beyond Good and Evil.* Translated by R. J. Hollingdale. Harmondsworth, UK: Penguin Books, 1973.

Owens, Lama Rod. *Love and Rage: The Path of Liberation through Anger.* Berkeley, CA: North Atlantic Books, 2020.

Parker, Dr. Gail. *Restorative Yoga for Ethnic and Race-Based Stress and Trauma.* London: Singing Dragon, 2020.

Purser, Ronald E. *McMindfulness: How Mindfulness Became the New Capitalist Spirituality.* London: Repeater Books, 2019.

Raheem, Octavia. *Gather.* Octavia Raheem, self-published, 2020.

Roundtree, Sage, and Alexandra Desiato. *Teaching Yoga Beyond the Poses: A Practical Workbook for Integrating Themes, Ideas, and Inspiration in Your Class.* Berkeley, CA: North Atlantic Books, 2019.

Salzberg, Sharon. *Real Change: Mindfulness to Heal Ourselves and the World.* New York: Flatiron Books, 2020.

Sanford, Matthew. *Waking: A Memoir of Trauma and Transcendence*. Emmaus, PA: Rodale, 2006.

Simpson, Daniel. *The Truth of Yoga: A Comprehensive Guide to Yoga's History, Texts, Philosophy, and Practices*. New York: North Point Press, 2021.

Singleton, Mark. *Yoga Body: The Origins of Modern Posture Practice*. Oxford: Oxford University Press, 2010.

Slatoff-Ponte, Zoe. *Yogavataranam: The Translation of Yoga*. New York: North Point Press, 2015.

Spindler, Beth. *Yoga Therapy for Fear: Treating Anxiety, Depression and Rage with the Vagus Nerve and Other Techniques*. London: Singing Dragon, 2018.

Stanley, Tracee, *Radiant Rest: Yoga Nidra for Deep Relaxation & Awakened Clarity*. Boulder: Shambhala Publications, 2021.

Stone, Michael. *The Inner Tradition of Yoga: A Guide to Yoga Philosophy for the Contemporary Practitioner*. Boston, MA: Shambhala Publications, 2008.

———. *Yoga for a World Out of Balance: Teachings on Ethics and Social Action*. Boston, MA: Shambhala Publications, 2009.

Swanson, Ann. *Science of Yoga: Understand the Anatomy and Physiology to Perfect Your Practice*. New York: DK Books, 2019.

Venkatesananda, Swami. *The Concise Yoga Vasistha*. Albany: State University of New York Press, 1984.

Wallis, Christopher D. *Tantra Illuminated: The Philosophy, History, and Practice of a Timeless Tradition*. Boulder, CO: Mattamayura Press, 2013.

Wijeyakumar, Anusha. *Meditation with Intention: Quick & Easy Ways to Create Lasting Peace*. Woodbury, MN: Llewellyn, 2021.

Wildcroft, Theodora. *Post-Lineage Yoga: From Guru to #MeToo*. Bristol, CT: Equinox Publishers, 2020.

Williams, Justin Michael. S*tay Woke: A Meditation Guide for the Rest of Us*. Boulder, CO: Sounds True, 2020.

williams, Rev. angel Kyodo, Lama Rod Owens, and Jasmine Syedullah, PhD. *Radical Dharma: Talking Race, Love, and Liberation*. Berkeley, CA: North Atlantic Books, 2016.

Yamasaki, Zahabiyah A. *Trauma-Informed Yoga for Survivors of Sexual Assault: Practices for Healing and Teaching with Compassion*. New York: W. W. Norton & Company, 2021.

Yang, Larry. *Awakening Together: The Spiritual Practice of Inclusivity and Community*. Somerville, MA: Widsom Publications, 2017.

# GLOSSARY

**ableism**—Discrimination based on disability. The false belief that some bodies (usually nondisabled bodies) are superior to other bodies.

**ACT UP**—AIDS Coalition To Unleash Power. This was a grassroots activist group that arose in response to the AIDS epidemic in the 1980s.

**ahamkara**—Can be defined as ego, or the storyteller in our head. The voice of the ego-mind.

**ahimsa**—The first of the five aspects of *yama*, the first limb of *ashtanga yoga*. *Ahimsa* means non-harm or nonviolence.

**aklishta**—Not causing suffering.

**aparigraha**—Nonattachment or non-greed.

**Arjuna**—The protagonist of the Bhagavad Gita. He is a great warrior and the leader of the Pandava brothers.

**asana**—Yoga posture or pose.

**ashtanga yoga**—The eight limbs of yoga as described in Patanjali's Yoga Sutras in sutra 2.29. These include *yama, niyama, asana, pranayama, pratyahara, dharana, dhyana,* and *samadhi.*

**Ashtanga Yoga**—This is the name of a specific school of yoga created by Patabhi Jois.

**asmita**—A Sanskrit word for ego, specifically the feeling of having a separate identity, or I-am-ness.

**asteya**—The third aspect of *yama*. *Asteya* means not stealing, or generosity.

**atman**—Refers to the individual spirit within each of us.

**Barkan, Ady**—A disability activist who has ALS, also known for his work on health care and other related social justice issues.

**Bhagavad Gita**—The great Indian scripture that is a part of the larger epic, the Mahabharata. The Gita tells the story of Arjuna being counseled by Krishna on how to be a yoga practitioner. Written approximately 2,000 years ago. It is a sacred text of Hinduism, or Sanatana Dharma. See the Resources section for recommended translations.

**bhakti yoga**—The devotional practices of yoga, such as mantra, *kirtan* (chanting), prayer, having a specific deity or image of the divine.

**Bikram Yoga**—A particular school of hot yoga created by Bikram Choudhury.

**Black Lives Matter**—A cultural revolution that arose in response to police brutality and the murder of Black people by the police.

**brahmacharya**—The fourth aspect of *yama*. The term *brahmacharya* traditionally meant celibacy, but is often translated in more contemporary times as conscious use of energy or resources.

**Brahmin**—The priest caste in India.

***Brihadaranyaka Upanishad***—One of the principle Upanishads created around 700 B.C.E.

**caste**—The caste system is a type of hereditary social stratification based on rigid social groups.

**chitta**—Term used by Patanjali to refer to the larger container of the mind.

**Crenshaw, Kimberlé**—Lawyer, civil rights advocate, and leading scholar on critical race theory.

**CrimethInc.**—A collective focused on representative democracy and radical community organizing. They create art and publish books, articles, and records.

**dharana**—The sixth limb of *ashtanga yoga*. *Dharana* means concentration, and is often described as the main practice of yoga meditation: focusing the mind on one thing.

**dhyana**—The seventh limb of *ashtanga yoga*. *Dhyana* means meditation, and describes the mental state that occurs in meditation, when the mind is connected to one focus.

**Dialectical Behavior Therapy** (**DBT**)—A type of psychotherapy developed by Marsha Linehan, PhD, as a modified form of cognitive behavior therapy. It focuses on skills for working with the mind.

**Duryodhana**—Arjuna's main opponent in the battle described in the Bhagavad Gita.

**Frankl, Viktor**—A psychologist who survived being a prisoner in the Nazi concentration camps during World War II and authored *Man's Search for Meaning*.

**Gayatri mantra**—An ancient and cherished mantra found in the Vedas.

**Girma, Haben**—A contemporary disability activist who is deaf-blind, graduated from Harvard Law School and worked in the Obama White House.

**gunas**—The three constituents of nature, or aspects of nature. They include *sattva*, *tamas*, and *rajas*.

**guru tattva**—The essence of the guru, or the divine principle.

**Hafiz**—A fourteenth-century Persian poet and mystic.

**Hanh, Thich Nhat**—A contemporary Vietnamese Buddhist monk who is known for his activism and social justice work. He founded the Plum Village Monastery in France.

**hatha yoga**—Refers to the physical practice of yoga.

**Heumann, Judith**—A contemporary disability activist, who is known as one of the founders of the modern disability rights movement. The film *Crip Camp* details her story.

**HIV/AIDS**—HIV (human immunodeficiency virus) is the virus that causes AIDS (acquired immunodeficiency syndrome). AIDS has been a pandemic since the 1980s and continues to affect hundreds of thousands of people around the world each year. Over 30 million people have died of AIDS since it was discovered.

**Integral Yoga**—The school of yoga founded in the United States by Swami Satchidananda, headquartered in Yogaville, Virginia.

**ishvarapranidhana**—The third aspect of *kriya yoga* and the fifth aspect of *yama*. Devotion or surrender to the god of your understanding.

**jnana yoga**—The wisdom practices of yoga, usually focused on self-inquiry.

**Kabir**—A fifteenth-century Indian mystic poet.

**karma**—Action and the result of action.

**karma yoga**—The path of selfless action often expressed through service and is sometimes called *seva*.

**klesha**—Mental affliction or obstacle

**klishta**—Causing suffering.

**Krishna**—The teacher of Arjuna in the Bhagavad Gita, who is an incarnation of God.

**kriya yoga**—The first sutra in the second book of the Yoga Sutras of Patanjali, which includes three aspects: *tapas, svadhyaya,* and *ishvarapranidhana.*

**Kundalini Yoga**—A school of yoga founded by Yogi Bhajan.

**Matsyendra**—An ancient saint and yogi who is considered the founder of *hatha yoga,* the physical practices.

**mycorrhiza**—The symbiotic relationship between plants and fungus.

**nirodha**—Restraint, calm, or stillness.

**niyama**—The second limb of *ashtanga yoga,* which means observances.

**Patanjali**—The author of the Yoga Sutras, a demigod whom much of the teaching of yoga is attributed to.

**post-lineage yoga**—A term coined by the researcher Theodora Wildcroft, which refers to community-based or peer learning in yoga.

**prakriti**—Nature.

**pranayama**—The fourth limb of *ashtanga yoga,* which means breathing practices, or the expansion of energy.

**pratipaksha bhavana**—Contemplating the opposite, or reflection on the painful outcome of negative thinking.

**pratyahara**—The fifth limb of *ashtanga yoga,* which means withdrawal of the senses.

**purusha**—Spirit or true self.

**Queer Nation**—An activist group started in the 1980s that focused on raising awareness of queer issues and queer rights. The group focused mainly on large public events and actions.

**raja yoga**—Historically meant the meditative goal of yoga, but often used as a synonym for the practice of Patanjali's yoga, or *ashtanga yoga*.

**rajas**—One of the *gunas*, refers to excited or active energy.

**Rig Veda**—One of the four main Vedas from approximately 1500 B.C.E. It includes the oldest known text in any Indo-European language.

**Roberts, Ed**—A leader in the disability rights movement and the founder of the Independent Living movement.

**Rumi**—The thirteenth-century Persian mystic and poet. The Order of the Whirling Dervishes was created by his son as his legacy.

**samadhi**—The eighth, and final, limb of *ashtanga yoga*, which means enlightenment, or super consciousness.

**samskara**—Mental impressions from past actions (*karma*) which influence future actions.

**santosha**—The second aspect of *niyama*, which means contentment.

**Satchidananda, Swami**—The founder of the school Integral Yoga.

**sattva**—One of the three *gunas* which means peaceful energy.

**satya**—The second aspect of *yama*, which means truthfulness.

**seva**—Service or *karma yoga*.

**shaucha**—The first aspect of *niyama*, which means purity.

**Shavasana**—The corpse pose, or relaxation pose.

**shakti**—Primordial cosmic energy.

**shruti**—Revealed teachings.

**Shiva**—Whose name means "the auspicious one," is part of the Hindu trinity of gods, including Brahma and Vishnu. He is called "the Destroyer."

**shramana**—Monks or ascetics.

**Sivananda, Swami**—An active teacher and writer who trained many of the teachers who brought yoga to the West including Swami Satchidananda and Swami Vishnu Devananda. He founded the Divine Life Society and the Yoga-Vedanta Forest Academy.

**Sivananda Vedanta Yoga**—The school of yoga founded by Swami Vishnu Devananda, and named for his teacher, Swami Sivananda.

**svadhyaya**—The second aspect of *kriya yoga*, and the fourth *niyama*, which means self-study, study of the Vedas, recitation of mantra, or recitation of the Vedas.

**tamas**—One of the three *gunas*, which means lethargic energy.

**tapas**—The first aspect of *kriya yoga*, and the third *niyama*, which means purification, discipline, asceticism, or learning from suffering.

**vairagya**—Nonattachment, or literally, "without color."

**Vedanta**—One of the six schools of Hindu philosophy, focusing on the teachings of the Upanishads.

**Vedas**—A large body of ancient Indian scripture, including some of the oldest texts written in an Indo-European language. There are four Vedas:

Rig Veda, Yajurveda, Samaveda, and Atharaveda, which are then each divided into four subsections including the Upanishads.

**vritti**—Thought and emotion, or the movement and disturbances of the mind.

**white supremacy**—The belief (and systems that support it) that white people are superior than other races. The beliefs that support systemic racism.

**yama**—The first limb of *ashtanga yoga*, which means abstention.

**Yoga Sutras of Patanjali** (*Patanjalayogashastra*)—The text that is often considered the leading source of information for yoga philosophy, although there is some debate about how that came to be. The text includes 195 aphorisms, or short lessons, on how to practice yoga and attain levels of enlightenment. It was written approximately 400 C.E. See the "Resources" section for recommendations of translations.

# NOTES

## CHAPTER 1: ANCIENT TEACHINGS, CONTEMPORARY PRACTICE

1. James Mallinson and Mark Singleton, *Roots of Yoga* (London: Penguin Classics, 2017), xvii.
2. Theodora Wildcroft, *Post-Lineage Yoga* (Bristol, CT: Equinox Publishers, 2020).
3. Joshua J. Mark, "The Vedas: Definition," Ancient History Encyclopedia, June 9, 2020, https://www.ancient.eu/The_Vedas/.
4. Sheena Sood, "Towards a Critical Embodiment of Decolonizing Yoga," *Race and Yoga Journal* 5, no.1 (2020).
5. Anjali Rao, "How Casteism Manifests in Yoga Spaces," *Yoga International*. Accessed April 9, 2021. https://yogainternational.com/article/view/how-casteism-manifests-in-yoga-spaces.
6. Swami Satchidananda, *The Yoga Sutras of Patanjali* (Yogaville, VA: Integral Yoga Publications, 2003), sutra 2.31.
7. Ephrat Livni, "Physics Explains Why Time Passes Faster as You Age," *Quartz*, January 8, 2019. https://qz.com/1516804/physics-explains-why-time-passes-faster-as-you-age.
8. Mallinson and Singleton, *Roots of Yoga*, 18.
9. Swami Satchidananda, *The Yoga Sutras of Patanjali*, sutra 2.42.
10. Kelley Palmer, "Dismantling White Supremacy and Redistributing Power in Yoga Spaces." *Accessible Yoga Podcast*, episode 2, www.accessibleyogatraining.com/blog/002.
11. https://implicit.harvard.edu/implicit/takeatest.html.
12. Human Dignity Trust website, "Map of Countries That Criminalize LGBT People," www.humandignitytrust.org/lgbt-the-law/map-of-criminalisation/.
13. Madeleine Carlisle, "Two Black Trans Women Were Killed in the U.S.

in the Past Week as Trump Revokes Discrimination Protections for Trans People," *Time*, June 13, 2020.

14. Isabella Grullon Paz and Maggie Astor, "Black Trans Women Seek More Space in the Movement They Helped Start," *New York Times*, June 27, 2020.

15. David Oliver and Rasha Ali, "Why We Owe Pride to Black Transgender Women Who Threw Bricks at Cops," *USA Today*, June 24, 2019.

16. Paulo Freire, *Pedagogy of the Oppressed* (London: Penguin Classics, 1993), 18.

17. Miriam Hernandez and Lisa Bartley, "Bikram Yoga Founder Bikram Choudhury Trapped in Mexico After Passport Seized; Fleet of CA Cars to Be Auctioned," ABC News, February 13, 2020.

18. Br. Shankara, "The Wizard of Oz According to Vedanta, Part 1," Vedanta Atlanta Website, October 16, 2016.

19. American Psychological Association Online Dictionary, https://dictionary.apa.org/confirmation-bias.

## CHAPTER 2: THE GOAL OF YOGA: CLEAR PERCEPTION

1. Oxford Languages Online Dictionary, https://languages.oup.com/google-dictionary-en/.

2. Jijith Nadumuri, *Aitareya Upanishad*, 3.1.1–2. http://naalanda.wikidot.com/u-mukhy:apana.

3. The Human Rights Campaign (designer)AMK1211 at en.wikipedia (this version), public domain, via Wikimedia Commons.

4. "Global HIV & AIDS Statistics—2020 Fact Sheet," UNAIDS website, www.unaids.org.

5. "Kimberlé Crenshaw on Intersectionality, More than Two Decades Later," Columbia Law School website, www.law.columbia.edu/news.

6. Edwin F. Bryant, *The Yoga Sutras of Patanjali: A New Edition, Translation, and Commentary* (New York: North Point Press, 2009), 169, sutra 2.1.

7. Lama Rod Owens, *Love and Rage: The Path of Liberation Through Anger* (Berkeley, CA: North Atlantic Books, 2020), 226.

8. Victor E. Frankl, *Man's Search for Meaning: An Introduction to Logotherapy* (New York: Simon & Shuster, 1984).

9. Bryant, *The Yoga Sutras of Patanjali*, sutra 2.15

10. Bryant, *The Yoga Sutras of Patanjali*, 203.

11. Ibram X. Kendi, Instagram post, October 17, 2020.

12. Shyam Ranganathan, *Patanjali's Yoga Sutra* (Haryana, India: Penguin Books, 2008), sutra 2.16.

13. The Krishna Path, "Did Quantam Physics Come from the Vedas?" Uplift Connect website, July 21, 2016.

14. Swami Satchidananda, *The Yoga Sutras of Patanjali*, 124, sutra 2.28.

15. The Linehan Institute website, https://linehaninstitute.org/.

## CHAPTER 3: CONNECTING TO THE SOURCE OF THE TEACHINGS

1. Zoe Slatoff-Ponte, *Yogavataranam: The Translation of Yoga*, North Point Press, 2015.

2. Kelly McGonigal, "Gayatri Mantra: The Yoga Chant You Need in Your Gratitude Practice," *Yoga Journal*, December 22, 2011.

3. Raja Ravi Varma (1848–1906), "Gayatri Mantra Personified as a Goddess," https://commons.wikimedia.org/wiki/File:Gayatri1.jpg.

4. Eknath Easwaran, *The Bhagavad Gita* (Tomales, CA: Nilgiri Press, 2007), sloka 10.32–39.

5. Swami *Vivekananda, The Complete Works of Swami Vivekananda* (Calcutta: Advaita Ashram, Sri Gauranga Press, 1915), 211.

## CHAPTER 4: EMBODYING THE EIGHT LIMBS OF YOGA

1. Edward J. Steele et al., "Cause of Cambrian Explosion – Terrestrial or Cosmic?" *Progress in Biophysics and Molecular Biology* 136 (August 2018): 3–23.

2. Swami Satchidananda, *The Living Gita: The Complete Bhagavad Gita* (New York: Henry Holt & Company, 1990), sloka 2.53.

3. Swami Satchidananda, *The Yoga Sutras of Patanjali*, sutra 2.29.

4. Shyam Ranganathan, *Accessible Yoga Podcast*, episode 8, www.accessible yogatraining.com/blog/008.

5. Bryant, *The Yoga Sutras of Patanjali*, sutras 2.33-34.

## CHAPTER 5: RAINBOW MIND: ENLIGHTENMENT TODAY

1. Nischala Joy Devi, *The Secret Power of Yoga* (New York: Three Rivers Press, 2007), 180.

2. Matthew Remski, *Threads of Yoga: A Remix of Patanjali's Sutras with Commentary and Reverie* (Self-published, 2012), 110–111.

3. brown, adrienne maree. *Emergent Strategy: Shaping Change, Changing Worlds* (Chico, CA: AK Press, 2017), 11.

4. Swami Hariharananda Aranya, *Yoga Philosophy of Patanjali* (Albany: State University of New York Press, 1983), sutra 3.3.

5. Holly Erin Copeland, "The Heart of Mind," *Medium*, March 26, 2020.

6. "Neurocardiology," Wikipedia, https://en.wikipedia.org/wiki/Neurocardiology.

7. Michael Stone, *Yoga for a World Out of Balance: Teachings on Ethics and Social Action* (Boston, MA: Shambhala Publications, 2009), 169.

8. Michelle Starr, "Study Maps the Odd Structural Similarities between the Human Brain and the Universe," *Science Alert*, November 17, 2020.

9. The Arbinger Institute, *The Anatomy of Peace: Resolving the Heart of Conflict* (San Francisco: Berrett-Koehler Publishers, 2020), 114–115.

10. Rev. angel Kyodo williams, Lama Rod Owens, and Jasmine Syedullah, PhD, *Radical Dharma: Talking Race, Love, and Liberation* (Berkeley, CA: North Atlantic Books, 2016), xxvii.

11. Daniel Ladinsky, *The Gift: Poems by Hafiz the Great Sufi Master* (New York: Penguin Group, 1999).

12. Stone, *Yoga for a World Out of Balance*, 167.

13. A. G. Mohan and Dr. Ganesh Mohan, *Hatha Yoga Pradipika* (Svastha Yoga, 2017) verse 1.12.

14. Martin Luther King Jr., "Nomination of Thich Nhat Hanh for the Nobel Peace Prize," January 25, 1967. www.hartford-hwp.com/archives/45a/025.html.

15. Thich Nhat Hanh, "Please Call Me by My True Names (song & poem)," Plum Village Website. June 3, 2020.

16. Sharon Salzberg, *Real Change: Mindfulness to Heal Ourselves and the World* (New York: Flatiron Books, 2020).

17. Swami Satchidananda, *The Living Gita*. sloka 2.48

18. www.malcolm-x.org/quotes.htm.

19. Lauren Frayer, "Gandhi Is Deeply Revered, but His Attitudes on Race and Sex Are Under Scrutiny," NPR, October 2, 2019.

20. Mohandas K. Gandhi, *The Bhagavad Gita According to Gandhi* (Berkeley, CA: Berkeley Hills Books, 2000), slokas 6:29–32.

21. Kirsch, Adam, "Modernity, Faith, and Martin Buber," *The New Yorker*, May 6, 2019.

22. Yogaville Closing Shlokas and Peace Chants, *Brihadaranyaka* and *Ishavasya Upanishads*, www.yogaville.org.

## CHAPTER 6: HONEST REFLECTION

1. Bryan Robinson, PhD, "New Study Shows Surprising Benefits of Yoga to Deal with Anxiety and Stress," *Forbes*, August 16, 2020.

2. Robert Bly, *The Soul Is Here for Its Own Joy*. page 85

3. https://www.elearningworld.org/i-i-knew-now-i-know-better-i-better/

4. Swami Satchidananda, *The Living Gita*, sloka 2.40.

## CHAPTER 7: DEATH IS THE ULTIMATE TEACHER

1. Swami Satchidananda, *The Yoga Sutras of Patanjali*, sutra 2.9.

2. Eknath Easwaran, *The Bhagavad Gita*, 21–22

3. Juan Mascaro, *The Bhagavad Gita* (London: Penguin Books, 1962), sloka 2.7–8.

4. Juan Mascaro, *The Upanishads* (London: Penguin Books, 1965), 57–59.

5. Eknath Easwaran, *The Bhagavad Gita*, sloka 2.20.

6. BJ Miller, "What Is Death: How the Pandemic Is Changing Our Understanding of Mortality," *New York Times*, December 20, 2020.

7. Owens, *Love & Rage*, 16.

8. Eknath Easwaran, *The Bhagavad Gita*, slokas 2.11–13, 16–18.

## CHAPTER 8: YOGA IS SERVICE

1. Eknath Easwaran, *The Bhagavad Gita*, sloka 3.25.

2. Ferris Jabr, "The Social Life of Forests: Trees Appear to Communicate and Cooperate through Subterranean Networks of Fungi. What Are They Sharing with One Another?" *New York Times*, December 2, 2020.

3. Ashley Spencer, "A Young Adult Author's Tweet Went Viral—But Somehow, Dr. Fauci Got the Credit," *Oprah*, August 26, 2020.

4. CrimethInc., "For All We Care: Reconsidering Self-Care," www.crimethinc.com.

5. Rachel Naomi Remen, "Helping, Fixing or Serving?" *Shambhala Sun*, September 1999.

6. Sara Rigby, "Rats Avoid Actions That Will Hurt Others—Even If It Earns Them a Treat," *Science Focus*, March 6, 2020.

## CHAPTER 9: PRACTICE IN REAL LIFE

1. German Lopez, "The Reagan Administration's Unbelievable Response to the HIV/AIDS Epidemic," *Vox*, December 1, 2016.

2. A pink triangle against a black backdrop with the words "Silence = Death," representing an advertisement for The Silence = Death Project, used by permission of ACT UP, the AIDS Coalition To Unleash Power

3. "Global HIV & AIDS Statistics—2020 Fact Sheet," UNAIDS website, www.unaids.org.

4. Reverend Jaganth Carrera, *Inside the Yoga Sutras* (Yogaville, VA: Integral Yoga Publications, 2006), 80.

5. Mascaro, *The Bhagavad Gita*, slokas 2:62–66.

6. Johnson, Michelle Cassandra, *Skill in Action: Radicalizing Your Yoga Practice to Create a Just World* (self-published 2017) 19–20.

7. Kevin Daum, "Inspiring Quotes from Michelle Obama," Inc.com.

## CHAPTER 10: THE EVOLUTION OF OUR PRACTICE

1. Kempton, Sally, "Yoga and Ego: Sophisticated Ego, How to Face Your Inner Self," *Yoga Journal*, August 25, 2007. https://www.yogajournal.com/yoga-101/philosophy/sophisticated-ego.

2. Bryant, *The Yoga Sutras of Patanjali*, sutra 2.6.

3. Bly, *The Soul Is Here for Its Own Joy*, 236

4. Pandit Rajmani Tigunait, *The Practice of the Yoga Sutra: Sadhana Pada* (Honesdale, PA: Himalayan Institue, 1998), 34.

5. See Heingartner, Douglas, "New Study Links Some Forms of Spiritual Training to Narcissism and 'Spiritual Superiority,'" *Psych News Daily*, November 29, 2020; and Kaufman, Scott Barry, "The Science of Spiritual Narcissism," *Scientific American*, January 11, 2021.

6. Caroline Delbert, "Animals Keep Evolving into Crabs, Which Is Somewhat Disturbing," *Popular Mechanics*, October 19, 2020.

## CHAPTER 11: ENGAGED YOGA

1. Swami Prabhavananda and Christopher Isherwood, *How to Know God: The Yoga Aphorisms of Patanjali* (Hollywood, CA: Vedanta Society, 1981), 150.
2. Death Penalty Information Center: Policy Issues, "Racial Bias against Defendants of Color and in Favor of White Victims Has a Strong Effect on Who Is Capitally Prosecuted, Sentenced to Death, and Executed," Deathpenaltyinfo.org.
3. Adam Liptak, "A Vast Racial Gap in Death Penalty Cases, New Study Finds," *New York Times*, August 3, 2020.
4. Larry Buchanan et al., "Black Lives Matter May Be the Largest Movement in U.S. History," *New York Times*, July 3, 2020.
5. Dr. Gail Parker, *Restorative Yoga for Ethnic and Race-Based Stress and Trauma* (London: Singing Dragon, 2020), 29.
6. Leslie Becker-Phelps, PhD, "Don't Just React: Choose Your Response," *Psychology Today*, July 23, 2013.
7. Swami Satchidananda, *The Living Gita*, sloka 2.70
8. Friedrich Nietzsche, *Beyond Good and Evil*, trans, R. J. Hollingdale (Harmondsworth, UK: Penguin Books, 1973); revised reprint 1990.
9. Swami Satchidananda, *The Living Gita*, sloka 3.4, 5, 8, 9.
10. M. K. Gandhi, *My Experiments with Truth* (London: Penguin Books, 2012), 435.
11. Dianne Bondy, "Yoga, Race, and Culture," *Yoga International*. Accessed April 9, 2021. https://yogainternational.com/article/view/yoga-race-and-culture

## CHAPTER 12: BUILDING COMMUNITY

1. Kevin C. Costley, PhD, "Research Supporting Integrated Curriculum: Evidence for Using This Method of Instruction in Public School Classrooms," February 1, 2015, https://files.eric.ed.gov.
2. Lisa M. Landreman, *The Art of Effective Facilitation: Reflections from Social Justice Educators* (Sterling, VA: Stylus Publishing, 2013).
3. The Nap Ministry website, https://thenapministry.wordpress.com/.
4. The HOMO being. "Shikhandi - a transgender | Shikhandi in Mahabharata | Who was Shikhandi in Mahabharata | English." On-

line video clip. YouTube. April 29, 2020. https://www.youtube.com /watch?v=UKXoiZpPRYs.

5. Diana Raab, PhD, "What Is Spiritual Bypassing?" *Psychology Today*, January 23, 2019.

6. Swami Satchidananda, *The Living Gita*, sloka 6.29–32

### SUMMARY OF PART TWO

1. Gandhi, Arun. *The Gift of Anger* (New York: Jeter Publishing, 2017) 18

### PART THREE: YOGA IN PRACTICE

1. Matthew Sanford, *Evolution of Yoga Summit Blueprint*, 2020 (Yoga Alliance conference journal article) https://www.yogaalliance.org/Get _Involved/COVID-19_Resources/

### CHAPTER 13: FINDING YOUR INNER TEACHER

1. Rasha Aridi, "Bird Flies 7,500 Miles, a New Record for Longest Nonstop Bird Migration," *Smithsonian*, October 16, 2020.

2. Swami Satchidananda, *The Yoga Sutras of Patanjali*, sutra 2.46.

3. Bryant, *The Yoga Sutras of Patanjali*, 287, sutra 2.47.

4. Elizabeth Quinn, "Visualization Techniques for Athletes," *Verywell Fit*, July 27, 2020.

### CHAPTER 14: CARING FOR YOURSELF WITH YOGA

1. Swami Satchidananda, *The Yoga Sutras of Patanjali*, 2.48.

### CHAPTER 15: A SAMPLE PRACTICE

1. Prayer Center, Satchidananda Ashram—Yogaville. https://www.yoga ville.org/discover/prayer-center/

### SUMMARY OF PART THREE

1. Mascaro, *The Upanishads*, 8.1.

# CONTRIBUTORS

**Adrian Molina** has been teaching yoga since 2004, with an extensive world-wide following through his platform and school of yoga, Warrior Flow. Adrian is also a writer, meditation teacher, sound therapist, end-of-life doula, mental health first-aid facilitator, ambassador for Accessible Yoga and Yoga for All, and soon to be TCTSY facilitator. Adrian is recognized as a community organizer and founder of the Warrior Flow Foundation, a 501(c)(3) nonprofit that brings the benefits of movement, therapeutic and accessible yoga, mindfulness, and stress reduction tools to schools, shelters, hospitals, police, first responders, and hospice care. He is also the cofounder of Warrior Flow TV, an online video platform that makes fitness and yoga accessible to anyone, anywhere, anytime. Find him at warriorflow.com.

**Amber Karnes** is a yoga teacher trainer, ruckus maker, the founder of Body Positive Yoga, and a lifelong student of her body. Amber trains yoga teachers and movement educators how to create accessible and equitable spaces for liberation and belonging. She also creates community for folks who want to build unshakable confidence and learn to live without shame or apology in the bodies they have today. Amber is the cocreator of the Accessible Yoga Training School and Yoga for All Teacher Training, Accessible Yoga Association board president, and a sought-after contributor on the topics of accessibility, authentic marketing, culture-shifting, and community building. She lives in Baltimore, Maryland, with her husband Jimmy. You can find her at bodypositiveyoga.com.

**Amina Naru, ERYT, YACEP,** is the owner of Posh Yoga LLC in Wilmington, Delaware, cofounder of Retreat to Spirit, active member of the board of directors for Accessible Yoga Association, and works as a trauma-sensitive yoga teacher, wellness educator, and workshop facilitator. Her professional expertise is in the field of yoga service for communities, juvenile detention centers, and adult prisons. She is the first black woman to implement curriculum-based yoga and mindfulness programs for juvenile detention centers in the state of Delaware. Amina is a contributor to the Best Practices book series for Yoga Service Council INC. and Omega Institute of Holistic Studies. She also served as project manager and contributor for *Yoga and Resilience: Empowering Practices for Survivors of Sexual Trauma* (Handspring, 2020). Amina is the cocreator of the *Yoga Journal* online course, "Yoga for Self Care," and has been featured in publications like *Yoga Therapy Today* and *Yoga Journal*. You can find her at posh-yoga.com.

**Anjali Rao** came to the yoga mat at nearly forty recovering from surgery from breast cancer. Growing up in Bangalore, India, karma and bhakti yoga were a way of life. She studies and teaches yoga philosophy/history from a sociopolitical perspective and is deeply interested in the intersectionality of race, culture, gender, and the accessibility of yoga practices. She aims to make the practice and study of yoga—on and off the mat—helpful and joyful to people across ages, genders, and abilities. She is a part of the faculty in various 200- and 300-hour teacher trainings in the country and considers herself a lifelong student. She serves on the board for HERS Breast Cancer Foundation, a nonprofit that helps survivors and those going through treatment regardless of financial status. Her website is yoganjali.me.

**De Jur Jones** has been a yoga devotee since 2001. She attended Loyola Marymount University's Yoga Therapy program. She teaches a therapeutic style of yoga suitable for most students. Along with having taught countless mainstream classes, De Jur offers programs and classes to incarcerated and formerly incarcerated people, unhoused populations, mentally challenged seniors, foster youth, those in recovery, human trafficking victims/survivors, and staff that serve all of these groups. De Jur is a contributor to the Yoga Service Council's "Best Practices for Yoga in the Criminal Justice System." She is an Accessible Yoga Ambassador and featured model in Jivana Heyman's book *Accessible Yoga, Poses and Practices for Every Body* and a yoga model for *Yoga After 50 for Dummies* by Dr. Larry Payne, PhD, and Melanie Klein's *Embodied Resilience through Yoga: 30 Mindful Essays*. De Jur cochaired at the 2019 International Association of Yoga Therapists Conference. De Jur moonlights as a flight attendant. Her website is idreaminyoga.com.

**Itzel Berrio Hayward** is a compassionate and fierce advocate for love. After serving as a public policy lawyer for thirteen years, Itzel left her legal career and founded Attuned Living, a mindfulness and wellness organization that helps individuals heal the sense of separation they feel from others—or even from themselves. Her unique work—based on the teachings of yoga, mindfulness, and compassionate communication—ranges from promoting social justice work within organizations and communities to guiding individuals on their search for personal and professional fulfillment. Today, Itzel holds retreats, classes, trainings, and private one-on-one sessions online, over the phone, and in person with people from all over the world. Her mission is to gently remind you of your individual wholeness and your interconnectedness with others and all of life. Her website is attunedliving.com.

**Jacquie "Sunny" Barbee** is an E-RYT 200-hour yoga teacher living in the panhandle of Florida. Sunny finished YTT in 2016 after turning to an asana practice to help with her chronic illness and depression. While in YTT she realized there was a need for more teachers that didn't fit the stereotypical "yoga body" image like her and that she could make a difference in helping people see that yoga is for every body. She is able to share with others how to customize their practice to fit their own body, whether that body is larger, aging, or living with illness or injury, much like she does with her practice. Creating safe spaces where the student can connect and make peace with their bodies is what Sunny loves most about teaching yoga. She is also certified in Accessible Yoga, Yoga for All Bodies, Mind Body Solutions, and Yin Yoga. Her website is sunnybeeyoga.net.

**Jonathan (J) Miles** is a yoga teacher who has been dancing to the rhythm of life since childhood. Yogi, martial artist, body worker, retired breakdancer, community activist, and the son of a Baptist minister, J Miles has been learning and studying Eastern arts and philosophy for nearly two decades. Creative self-expression and exploration of the self through movement have always been a constant source of curiosity and confidence. Over the years J has crafted a style tempered by real life and humor that relies on the importance of breath as a guide and a source of strength. His classes aim to create for each person a fluid, sustainable, and enjoyable practice that hopefully will prove to be beneficial over a lifetime. And even as this ancient practice continues to evolve, the mantra continues to be "practice is effort toward steadiness of mind." His website is mahavirarva.com.

**Marc Settembrino** is a fat-queer educator, researcher, and yoga facilitator based in Hammond, Louisiana. Marc envisions a world that celebrates diversity and promotes dignity. In 2018, Marc created Fat Kid Yoga Club, a supportive yoga community for folks with larger bodies to explore joyful movement and celebrate what is possible in their bodies one practice at a time. Fat Kid Yoga Club is a truly judgment-free zone where folks like Marc, who were always picked last or have experienced a lifetime of body shame, get to reconnect with their bodies and have fun at the same time. Their website is fatkidyogaclub.com.

**Mei Lai Swan.** Born on the unceded indigenous lands of Australia, Mei Lai Swan is the founder of the social enterprise yoga school Yoga for Humankind, offering specialized trainings in Trauma-Informed Yoga and Embodied Social Change. Dedicated to the paths of yoga, meditation, and community practice for over twenty years, Mei Lai Swan's approach to yoga is deeply embodied, inclusive, and inquiry-based. She is an experienced yoga teacher trainer and certified Embodied Flow facilitator with a professional background in music, community development, and social work. Mei Lai specializes in trauma-informed yoga and social justice, somatics, and nada yoga (sound and mantra). Mei Lai is passionate about building community and making the richness and depth of the yoga teachings and practices accessible, relevant, and empowering for every body, heart, and mind. Her website is yogaforhumankind.org.

**Melanie "M" Camellia** (they/them) is a fat, queer, nonbinary, neuroemergent yoga teacher, writer, and advocate, called to create profoundly accessible spaces for self-inquiry. They believe that the goal of yoga is collective liberation and challenge contemporary yoga practitioners to dismantle the systems and beliefs that hold us all back. M is a cofounder of the Trans Yoga Project and serves on the staff of Accessible Yoga, among other roles within the realm of yoga service. Their teaching and writing often center Queer and Trans* identity, consent and agency, fat liberation, and disability justice in relation to yoga philosophy and practice, and they serve as a mentor for other yoga teachers and practitioners desiring to deepen their understanding of accessibility, trauma, and yoga as social justice. M lives in Silver Spring, Maryland, with two cat companions, Matcha and Chai, and regularly teaches online and in the Washington, DC, metro area. Their website is mcamellia.com.

**Michelle Cassandra Johnson** is an author, yoga teacher, social justice activist, intuitive healer, and dismantling racism trainer. She approaches her life and work from a place of empowerment, embodiment, and integration. As a dismantling racism trainer, she has worked with large corporations, nonprofits, and community groups, including the ACLU-WA, Duke University, Google, *This American Life*, Eno River Unitarian Universalist Church, Lululemon, and many others. Michelle published *Skill in Action: Radicalizing Your Yoga Practice to Create a Just World* in 2017; she teaches workshops in yoga studios and community spaces nationwide. Michelle's new book, *Finding Refuge: Heart Work for Healing Collective Grief*, published by Shambhala Publications, July 2021. Whether in an anti-oppression training, yoga space, individual or group intuitive healing session, the heart, healing, and wholeness are at the center of how Michelle approaches all of her work in the world. Her website is michellecjohnson.com.

**Octavia Raheem** is a mother, author of *Gather*, yoga teacher, and founder of Starshine & Clay Online Yoga and Meditation Studio for Black Women and Women of Color. Octavia is a deep listener and a truth teller. She is a gatherer and space holder for rest and awakening. As a teacher and leader she has the skill of hearing beneath the surface for what isn't being said, yet needs to be. She guides us toward resonance and connection even when the truths we witness, hear, and encounter vary from our own. Octavia has more than fifteen years of experience and nearly 10,000 hours of leading classes, immersions, and trainings. She has studied with Dr. Gail Parker (Restorative Yoga), Tracee Stanley (Yoga Nidra), Chanti Tacoronte Perez (Yoga Nidra and Restorative Yoga), Maya Breuer (The Art of Holding Space), Graham Fowler (200 hour), Yoganand Michael Carroll (Advanced

Studies), and Gina Minyard (Sacred Alignment and Anatomy). She is proud to call them her teachers. Her website is octaviaraheem.com.

**Rane Bowen** (he/him) is a longtime student of yoga and meditation. He has an insatiable curiosity about these practices and how they can help people in their daily lives and in overcoming adversity. Rane's interest in these practices deepened after being diagnosed with stomach cancer and subsequently having his stomach removed in 2015. He found these practices helped him cope with the emotional difficulties of a terminal (mis) diagnosis and aided in his recovery. Rane teaches yoga at Garden of Yoga, a home-based studio he runs with his wife and partner Jo Stewart. Together they host the *Flow Artists Podcast*, in which they speak to teachers and thinkers about yoga, meditation, social justice, and more. You can find them at podcast.flowartists.com.

**Sarit Z. Rogers** is a Somatic Experiencing Practitioner, accomplished photographer, writer, group facilitator, and trauma-informed yoga teacher. Sarit's yoga certifications include a 200-hour trauma-informed Hatha/Vinyasa, Accessible Yoga, Yoga for All, Restorative and Yin yoga. Sarit facilitates groups and provides Somatic Experiencing sessions to adolescents and adults in treatment. Sarit integrates mindfulness, invitational language, movement, and self-awareness, encouraging students to develop accessible tools for self-care, self-regulation, and healthy boundaries. Her goal is to bring yoga and SE to underserved communities where healing is needed the most and is often out of reach. Sarit is currently assisting Somatic Experiencing trainings, as well as participating in multiple advanced SE trainings to deepen and broaden her abilities to promote wellness. To contact Sarit regarding writing, yoga and Somatic Experiencing, see saritzrogers.com and for photography, see saritphotography.com.

**Susanna Barkataki.** An Indian yoga practitioner in the Shankaracharya tradition, Susanna Barkataki supports practitioners to lead with equity, diversity and yogic values while growing thriving practices and businesses with confidence. She is founder of Ignite Yoga and Wellness Institute and runs 200/500 Yoga Teacher Training programs. She is an E-RYT 500, Certified Yoga Therapist with International Association of Yoga Therapists

(C-IAYT). Author of the #1 New Release and International Bestseller in Yoga in November 2020, *Embrace Yoga's Roots: Courageous Ways to Deepen Your Yoga Practice*. With an honors degree in philosophy from UC Berkeley and a master's in education from Cambridge College, Barkataki is a diversity, accessibility, inclusivity, and equity (DAIE) yoga unity educator who created the groundbreaking Honor {Don't Appropriate} Yoga Summit with over 10,000 participants. Learn more and take her complimentary masterclass to embrace yoga's roots without appropriation at namastemasterclass.com.

## PHOTO CREDITS

All images of Jivana Heyman by Sarit Z. Rogers Photography
Susanna Barkataki by Eran James, Ignite Yoga and Wellness Institute
Michelle Cassandra Johnson by DesiLui Photography
Jonathan (J) Miles by Daniel Ewing
Anjali Rao by Yatin Rao
Jacquie "Sunny" Barbee by Anabel T. Barbee
Amber Karnes by John Robinson
Sarit Z. Rogers by De Jur Jones
Amina Naru by Herman Vandebrandt
Rane Bowen by Danielle Lara Woolley, This Wild Soul Photography
De Jur Jones by Sarit Z. Rogers Photography
Adrian Molina by Sway Photos
Octavia Raheem by LeeAnn Chisolm Morrissette
Itzel Berrio Hayward self-portrait
Mei Lai Swan by Emma Louise Costabile
Marc Settembrino by Tammie Quintana
M Camellia by Jordan Battiste